Pulmonary Physiology and Pathophysiology

An Integrated, Case-Based Approach

Pulmonary Physiology and Pathophysiology

An Integrated, Case-Based Approach

John B. West, M.D., Ph.D., D.Sc.

Professor of Medicine and Physiology
University of California, San Diego
School of Medicine
La Jolla, California

LIPPINCOTT WILLIAMS & WILKINS
A **Wolters Kluwer** Company

Philadelphia · Baltimore · New York · London
Buenos Aires · Hong Kong · Sydney · Tokyo

Editor: Robert Anthony
Managing Editor: Jacquelyn Merrell
Marketing Manager: Aimee Sirmon
Production Editor: Bill Cady

351 West Camden Street
Baltimore, Maryland 21201-2436 USA

530 Walnut Street
Philadelphia, Pennsylvania 19106-3621 USA

The publisher is not responsible (as a matter of product liability, negligence, or otherwise) for
any injury resulting from any material contained herein. This publication contains
information relating to general principles of medical care which should not be construed as
specific instructions for individual patients. Manufacturers' product information and package
inserts should be reviewed for current information, including contraindications, dosages, and
precautions.

Printed in the United States of America

Library of Congress Cataloging-in-Publication Data

West, John B.
  Pulmonary physiology and pathophysiology : an integrated, case-based approach / John B.
West—1st ed.
     p. cm.
  Includes index.
  ISBN 0-7817-2910-6
     1. Respiratory organs—Pathophysiology—Case studies. 2. Respiratory organs—
Physiology—Case studies. I. Title.
  RC711 .W47 2000
  616.2′0047—dc21

                                                            00-056542

*The publishers have made every effort to trace the copyright holders for borrowed material. If they
have inadvertently overlooked any, they will be pleased to make the necessary arrangements at the
first opportunity.*

To purchase additional copies of this book call our customer service department at **(800)
638-3030** or fax orders to **(301) 824-7390**. International customers should call **(301)
714-2324**.

Lippincott Williams & Wilkins customer service representatives are available from 8:30 am
to 6:00 pm, EST, Monday through Friday, for telephone access. Or *visit Lippincott Williams
& Wilkins on the Internet:* **http://www.lww.com.**

                                                    00 01 02 03
                                                    1 2 3 4 5 6 7 8 9 10

Preface

A sound knowledge of the physiology and pathophysiology of the lung will always be necessary in clinical medicine because of the high prevalence of lung disease and the fact that optimal treatment is so closely related to an understanding of lung function. Traditionally, pulmonary physiology and pathophysiology have been taught as separate courses, often in the first and second years of medical school, respectively. Physiology is frequently linked with anatomy, and pathophysiology with pathology. This pattern has stood the test of time, and my two short textbooks, *Respiratory Physiology— The Essentials*, sixth edition, and *Pulmonary Pathophysiology—The Essentials*, fifth edition, were written for such courses and have been extensively used.

Recently, an increasing number of medical schools have experimented with integrating the two courses. There are several pressures to do this. One is the burgeoning advances in other preclinical sciences, especially molecular biology and medicine. These deserve additional attention in the preclinical years and therefore squeeze the time available for physiology. Another is the understandable desire of first-year medical students to see the relevance of what is being taught. We may *say* that dynamic compression of the airways is important in chronic obstructive pulmonary disease, but the student only realizes this when he or she learns how it causes disability in a patient. Finally, an integrated course introduces the student to clinical problems early and so piques his or her interest.

This book is written around seven case histories of patients with "bread and butter" diseases: chronic obstructive pulmonary disease, asthma, diffuse interstitial pulmonary fibrosis, pulmonary embolism, pulmonary edema, coal workers' pneumoconiosis, and acute respiratory failure. These follow two chapters on healthy subjects—both first-year medical students. Ann is a competitive cyclist, and Bill an avid mountaineer. These allow the necessary introduction of some of the principles of normal physiology. The book is focused on pulmonary physiology

and pathophysiology but includes some anatomy, pharmacology, and pathology. Much of the text is based on my other two books; in fact, in some respects the new book is a synthesis of these two books. Once you have decided on the best way to describe the oxygen dissociation curve, there is little point in trying to reinvent the wheel.

A new book like this raises the question of how much pulmonary physiology and pathophysiology a medical student should be taught, or more to the point, how much should he or she be expected to know. The answer is probably less material than 25 years ago, when the first edition of *Respiratory Physiology—The Essentials* appeared. At that time, molecular medicine was in its infancy, and nobody had envisaged sequencing the human genome. It is self-evident that as essential new material enters the preclinical curriculum, some material has to go. This new book covers about 90% of the material in the first nine chapters of *Respiratory Physiology—The Essentials* (the last chapter on "Tests of Pulmonary Function" was never intended to be part of the core material). The present book also includes about 70% of the material in parts II and III of *Pulmonary Pathophysiology—The Essentials*. (Part I is, to a large extent, a review of normal physiology.) In other words, expectations have been lowered, but the new book should certainly provide an adequate foundation for future learning in the clinical and post-M.D. years.

This book also raises some interesting didactic questions. The traditional courses allow the student to proceed logically from first principles. Normal physiology is covered first, and for example, the pathway of oxygen can be traced through ventilation, diffusion across the blood-gas barrier, pulmonary blood flow, carriage of oxygen by the blood, and blood-tissue gas exchange. This can be called teaching in series. By contrast, an integrated course develops topics in parallel and tends to be recursive or elliptical. A clinical case is introduced and prompts physiological questions; the answers may not always follow logically from what has already been learned. There are loose ends that have to be gathered up subsequently. Some students find this frustrating, while others are stimulated by the early clinical exposure.

However, the traditional "serial" approach is less logical in practice than it may seem to be. All of us have to return repeatedly to earlier concepts to review them. The notion that once a topic has been covered in detail, the resulting knowledge is firmly in place, is clearly a fallacy. We spend our professional lives going back to review earlier material, much of which was presented to us for the first time many years ago.

Many people have helped with this book. I would particularly like to thank Paul Kelly and Timothy Satterfield of Lippincott Williams & Wilkins, who identified the need for a book along these lines. Amy Clay provided invaluable help in the preparation of the manuscript. Much of the material has been modified over the years in response to discussions with our superb medical students at the University of California San Diego.

Contents

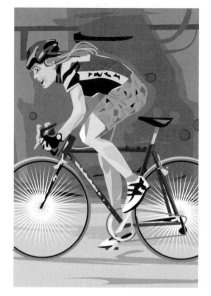

Chapter 1

Normal Physiology: Exercise

☐ In this chapter we meet Ann, a first-year medical student and competitive cyclist. She has a high maximal oxygen uptake, and we discuss the physiological processes that make this possible. These include pulmonary ventilation, diffusion of oxygen across the blood-gas barrier, pulmonary blood flow, carriage of oxygen by the blood, and diffusion of oxygen to the peripheral tissues.

☐ ABOUT ANN

Meet Ann, aged 23 years, a first-year medical student and competitive cyclist. She is healthy in all respects and has never had a serious illness. In addition to being a strong student who majored in biology in college and received excellent grades, Ann is an outstanding athlete. She became interested in competitive cycling while in high school, and in college she successfully competed at the national level. Although she is now too busy to train at the required level for competition, she rides every day and keeps herself very fit.

Ann had a medical examination before coming to medical school, and no abnormalities were found. At that time a chest radiograph was normal, and a blood test showed a hemoglobin concentration of $14 \ g \cdot dl^{-1}$.

Because of her interest in exercise, Ann volunteered for a measurement of maximal oxygen uptake ($\dot{V}_{O_2}$max) in the pulmonary function laboratory using a stationary bicycle ($\dot{V}_{O_2}$ means volume of oxygen per unit time). The bicycle ergometer allowed the work rate (or power) to be increased gradually while Ann was pedaling. The results of the study are shown in **FIGURE 1–1A**. First, Ann's oxygen consumption ($\dot{V}_{O_2}$) was measured while she was at rest (work rate of zero). This was done by measuring with a flowmeter the amount of air she exhaled and determining

its concentrations of oxygen and carbon dioxide. Then Ann's work rate was gradually increased, and it can be seen that the $\dot{V}_{O_2}$ was linearly related to work rate. Eventually the $\dot{V}_{O_2}$ flattened out at a value defined as the $\dot{V}_{O_2}$max. In Ann's case this was $3.5 \ l \cdot min^{-1}$. Any increase in work rate above this level can only occur through anaerobic glycolysis, which does not utilize oxygen.

Figure 1–1B shows additional measurements that were made during Ann's exercise test. The volume of expired gas per minute (total ventilation [$\dot{V}_E$]) increased linearly with $\dot{V}_{O_2}$ up to a certain point and then increased more rapidly. If there is a clear inflection point, this is sometimes called the anaerobic threshold, although the term is somewhat controversial. The blood lactate concentration (*La*) often rises markedly above this point. Someone like Ann (who is very fit) can exercise to high work levels before producing much lactate, but less fit people develop increased blood lactate levels earlier. Figure 1–1B also shows Ann's cardiac output (Q̇). This is a more difficult measurement to make, but reasonably accurate values can be obtained by a rebreathing technique in which the rate of uptake of a soluble gas such as acetylene from the lung is determined.

Note the very large changes in the variables with exercise. $\dot{V}_{O_2}$ increased from 300 to 3500 $ml \cdot min^{-1}$ while total ventilation increased from

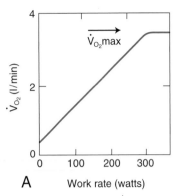

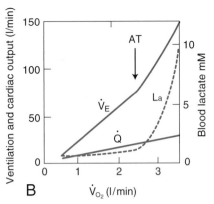

A

B

FIGURE 1–1. A. O_2 consumption ($\dot{V}_{O_2}$) increases nearly linearly with work rate until the $\dot{V}_{O_2}$max is reached. **B.** Ventilation ($\dot{V}_E$) initially increases linearly with O_2 consumption but rises more rapidly when substantial amounts of blood lactate (*La*) are formed. If there is a clear break, this is sometimes called the anaerobic threshold (*AT*). Cardiac output increases less than ventilation.

about 10 to 150 $1 \cdot min^{-1}$. By contrast, the cardiac output increased much less, from about 5 to 25 $1 \cdot min^{-1}$. Blood lactate rose from about 1 to 10 mM.

How is Ann able to raise her metabolic rate so much? The answer to this question allows us to be introduced to many aspects of normal pulmonary function. Let's look in turn at the various processes that allow Ann to have such a high oxygen consumption. This involves a coordinated set of physiological events including ventilation which gets gas to the alveoli, diffusion which enables oxygen to cross the blood-gas barrier, pulmonary blood flow which moves the oxygenated blood out of the lung, the transport of oxygen by the blood, and finally its diffusion to the mitochondria where the energy-producing reactions occur.

☐ VENTILATION: HOW GAS GETS TO THE ALVEOLI

Muscles of Respiration

Inspiration

The most important muscle of inspiration is the *diaphragm*, which is a thin, dome-shaped sheet of muscle attached to the lower ribs and spine. When Ann is cycling at high speed, this muscle contracts vigorously and moves downward like a piston **(FIGURE 1–2A)** with an excursion of as much as 10 cm, compared with only 1 cm during resting breathing. In this way, the vertical dimension of the chest cavity is increased, and the abdominal contents are forced downward and forward (Fig. 1–2B). In addition, the rib margins are lifted and moved out, thus increasing the transverse diameter of the thorax (Fig. 1–2A). The diaphragm is innervated by the two phrenic nerves that originate from cervical segments 3, 4, and 5 high in the neck. If one of these nerves is damaged, half of the diaphragm is paralyzed, and it moves up rather than down with inspiration because the intrathoracic pressure falls. This is known as *paradoxical movement*.

The *external intercostal muscles* connect adjacent ribs and slope downward and forward **(FIGURE 1–3A)**. When they contract, the ribs are pulled upward and forward, causing an increase in both the lateral and anteroposterior diameters of the thorax (Fig. 1–3B). The lateral dimension increases because of the "bucket-handle" movement of the ribs. The intercostal muscles are supplied by intercostal nerves that come off the spinal cord at the same level. Paralysis of the intercostal muscles alone does not seriously affect breathing because the diaphragm is so effective.

The *accessory muscles of inspiration* include the scalene muscles in the neck which elevate the first two ribs, and the sternomastoids which raise the sternum. There is little if any activity in these muscles during quiet breathing, but when Ann is pedaling hard, they can be seen to contract vigorously. Other muscles that are used during exercise include the alae nasi, which cause flaring of the nostrils, and small muscles in the neck and head.

Expiration

This is passive during quiet breathing because the lung and chest wall are elastic and tend to return to their equilibrium positions after being actively expanded during inspiration. However, when Ann is exercising hard, expiration is very active. The most important muscles are those of the *abdominal wall*, including the rectus abdominus, internal and external oblique muscles, and transversus abdominus. When these muscles contract, intra-abdominal pressure is raised, and the diaphragm is pushed upward (Fig. 1–2B). They also contract forcefully during coughing, vomiting, and defecation.

The *internal intercostal muscles* assist active expiration by pulling the ribs downward and inward, that is opposite to the action of the external intercostal muscles (Fig. 1–3A) thus decreasing the thoracic volume. In addition, they stiffen the intercostal spaces to prevent these from bulging outward during straining. It

should be added that the actions of respiratory muscles, especially the intercostals, are more complex than this brief account suggests.

Airways

The airways of the lung consist of a series of branching tubes which become narrower, shorter, and more numerous as they penetrate deeper into the lung (**FIGURE 1–4**). The trachea divides into right and left main bronchi, which in turn divide into lobar, then segmental bronchi. This process continues down to the *terminal bronchioles* which are the smallest airways without alveoli. All these bronchi make up the conducting airways. Their function is to lead inspired air to the gas-exchanging regions of the lung (**FIGURE 1–5**). Since the conducting airways contain no alveoli and therefore take no part in gas exchange, they constitute the *anatomic dead space*. Its volume is about 150 ml.

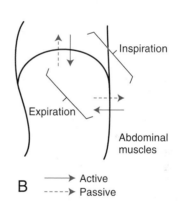

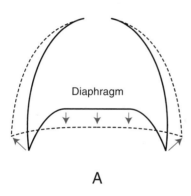

FIGURE 1–2. A. On inspiration, the dome-shaped diaphragm contracts, the abdominal contents are forced down and forward, and the rib cage is lifted. The volume of the thorax is therefore increased. **B.** On forced expiration, the abdominal muscles contract and push the diaphragm up.

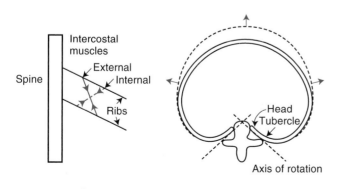

FIGURE 1–3. A. When the external intercostal muscles contract, the ribs are pulled upward and forward. **B.** The external intercostal muscles rotate on an axis joining the tubercle and head of the rib. As a result, both the lateral and anteroposterior diameters of the thorax increase. The internal intercostals have the opposite action.

The terminal bronchioles divide into *respiratory bronchioles* which have occasional alveoli budding from their walls. Finally, we come to the *alveolar ducts* which are completely lined with alveoli. This alveolated region of the lung where gas exchange occurs is known as the *respiratory zone*. The portion of the lung distal to a terminal bronchiole forms an anatomical unit called the *acinus*. The distance from the terminal bronchiole to the most distant alveolus is only a few millimeters, and the gas moves through this short distance chiefly by diffusion. The respiratory zone makes up most of the lung, its volume being about 2.5 to 3 liters.

It is important to distinguish between total ventilation ($\dot{V}_E$) and alveolar ventilation ($\dot{V}_A$). The latter is defined as the volume of *fresh* gas reaching the alveoli per minute. We saw (Fig. 1–1B) that Ann's total ventilation was determined by measuring the volume of the expired gas per unit time. This is very nearly equal to the volume of inspired gas. However, as **FIGURE 1–6**

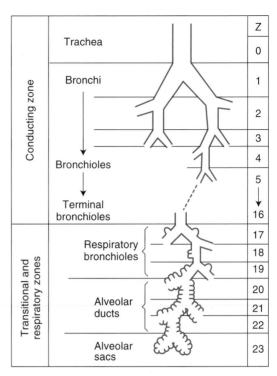

FIGURE 1–5. Idealization of the human airways according to Weibel. The first 16 generations (*Z*) make up the conducting airways, and the last 7 compose the respiratory zone (or the transitional and respiratory zone).

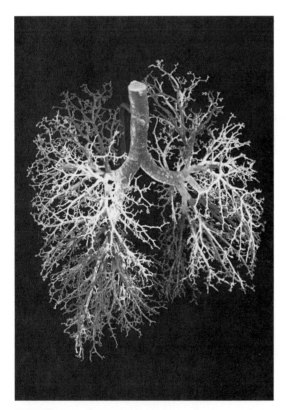

FIGURE 1–4. Cast of the airways of a human lung. The alveoli have been pruned away, allowing the conducting airways from the trachea to the terminal bronchioles to be seen.

indicates, not all of the total inspired volume per breath (tidal volume) gets to the alveoli. A portion remains in the anatomic dead space and is exhaled with the next expiration. Therefore, Ann's alveolar ventilation is the (tidal volume – anatomic dead space) × respiratory frequency.

☐ DIFFUSION: HOW GAS GETS ACROSS THE BLOOD-GAS BARRIER

Blood-Gas Barrier

The pulmonary capillaries are in the walls of the alveoli, and the blood-gas barrier is exceedingly thin (**FIGURE 1–7**). In fact, approximately half of the area of the barrier has a thickness of only 0.2 to 0.3 µm, whereas the total area of the barrier is as large as 50 to 100 m². This combination of extreme thinness and large area is ideal for diffusion.

The blood-gas barrier has only three layers: the alveolar epithelium (EP), capillary endothe-

VOLUMES   **FLOWS**

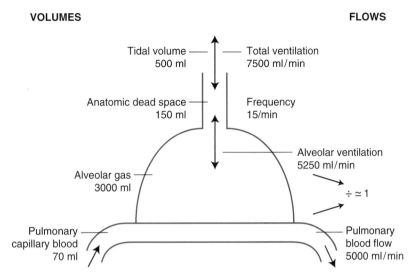

FIGURE 1–6. Diagram of a lung showing typical volumes and flows under resting conditions. There are considerable variations around these values.

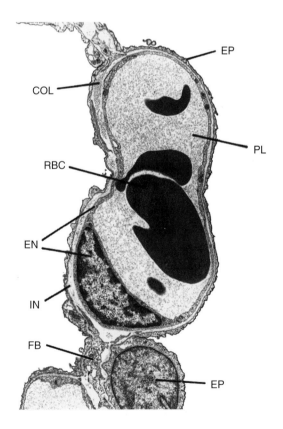

FIGURE 1–7. Electron micrograph showing a pulmonary capillary in the alveolar wall. Note the extremely thin blood-gas barrier, which is only 0.2 to 0.3 μm thick in some places. Oxygen diffuses from alveolar gas to the interior of the erythrocyte (*RBC*), and its path includes the layer of surfactant (not shown in the preparation), alveolar epithelium (*EP*), interstitium (*IN*), capillary endothelium (*EN*), and plasma (*PL*). Parts of structural cells called fibroblasts (*FB*), the nucleus of an endothelial cell (*EN*), and fibrils of type I collagen (*COL*) in the thick side of the blood-gas barrier are also seen.

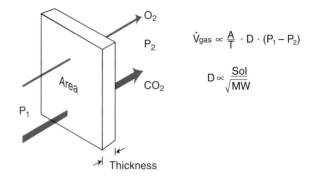

FIGURE 1–8. Diffusion through a tissue sheet. The amount of gas transferred is proportional to the area (A), a diffusion constant (D), and the difference in partial pressure (P$_1$–P$_2$), and is inversely proportional to the thickness (T). The constant is proportional to the gas solubility (Sol) but inversely proportional to the square root of the molecular weight (MW).

lium (EN), and interstitium (IN) sandwiched between them (Fig. 1–7). Many capillaries have a very thin blood-gas barrier on one side but a thicker barrier on the other where the IN is widened (Fig. 1–7). This thicker side is important for fluid exchange (*see* Chapter 7). Much of the barrier is so thin that if the pressure within the capillaries rises to abnormally high levels, or the tension in the alveolar wall is greatly increased by inflating the lung to a very high volume, the barrier can be damaged.

Principles of Diffusion

All gases pass across the blood-gas barrier by simple diffusion. Fick's law **(FIGURE 1–8)** states that the rate of transfer of a gas through a sheet of tissue is proportional to the tissue area (A) and the difference in gas partial pressure* between the two sides (P$_1$ – P$_2$), and inversely proportional to the tissue thickness (T). In addition, the rate of transfer is proportional to a diffusion constant (D) which depends on the properties of the tissue and the particular gas. The constant is proportional to the solubility (Sol) of the gas and inversely proportional to the square root of the molecular weight (MW). This means that CO_2 diffuses about 20 times more rapidly than O_2 through tissue sheets because it has a much higher Sol but not a very different MW.

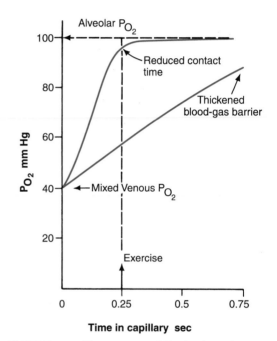

FIGURE 1–9. Time course of P$_{O_2}$ in the pulmonary capillary as O_2 is loaded. Under normal conditions the P$_{O_2}$ of capillary blood almost reaches that of alveolar gas within one-third of the time available. However, on exercise when pulmonary blood flow is greatly increased, the time available for loading the oxygen is greatly reduced. When the blood-gas barrier is thickened, the capillary P$_{O_2}$ rises more slowly because the diffusion rate of O_2 is slowed.

Oxygen Uptake Along the Pulmonary Capillary

FIGURE 1–9 shows how the P$_{O_2}$ rises as the blood loads oxygen in the pulmonary capillary. Under resting conditions, the blood spends only about 0.75 sec in the capillary; when Ann is exercising hard, this may be reduced to as little as 0.25 sec. During resting conditions the blood entering the lung has a P$_{O_2}$ of 40 mm Hg, and

---

* The partial pressure of a gas is found by multiplying its concentration by the total pressure. For example, dry air has 20.93% O_2. Its partial pressure (P$_{O_2}$) at sea level (barometric pressure 760 mm Hg) is therefore 20.93/100 × 760 = 159 mm Hg. When air is inhaled into the upper airways, it is warmed and moistened, and the water vapor pressure is then 47 mm Hg, so that the total dry gas pressure is only 760 − 47 = 713 mm Hg. The P$_{O_2}$ of inspired air is therefore 20.93/100 × 713 = 149 mm Hg. A liquid exposed to a gas until equilibration takes place has the same partial pressure as the gas. These topics are discussed more fully in Chapter 2. For a more complete description of the gas laws, see Appendix A.

since the P_{O_2} in alveolar gas is 100 mm Hg, oxygen floods down this large pressure gradient, and the P_{O_2} in the blood rapidly rises. Indeed it has almost reached the alveolar P_{O_2} after 0.25 sec. If the blood-gas barrier is thickened by disease and diffusion is therefore slowed, the P_{O_2} rises more slowly. We shall see a patient in which this occurs in Chapter 5.

Under resting conditions, Figure 1–9 shows that there is ample time for the P_{O_2} in the blood to virtually equilibrate with that in the alveolar gas. This means that the amount of oxygen taken up is determined by the amount of blood flow available. However, when Ann exercises at maximal intensity, the P_{O_2} in the blood only just reaches that of alveolar gas. Indeed in some elite athletes, equilibration fails to occur, and under these conditions, oxygen uptake is partly *diffusion limited*. If the blood-gas barrier is thickened (Fig. 1–9), diffusion limitation may even occur at rest and will be exaggerated on exercise.

□ PULMONARY BLOOD FLOW: HOW OXYGEN IS TRANSPORTED FROM THE LUNG

Blood Vessels

The pulmonary circulation begins at the main pulmonary artery, which receives the mixed venous blood pumped by the right ventricle **(FIGURE 1–10)**. This artery then branches successively like the system of airways (Figs. 1–4 and 1–5), and indeed the pulmonary arteries accompany the bronchi down the center of the lobules as far as the terminal bronchioles.

Beyond that they break up to supply the capillary bed which lies in the walls of the alveoli **(FIGURES 1–11 and 1–12)**. The dense network of capillaries in the alveolar walls is an exceedingly efficient arrangement for gas exchange. The oxygenated blood is then collected from the capillary bed by small pulmonary veins that run between the lobules and eventually unite to form the large veins that drain into the left atrium.

Pressures Inside and Outside the Pulmonary Blood Vessels

The pressures *within* the pulmonary circulation are remarkably low. The mean pressure in the main pulmonary artery is only about 15 mm Hg; the systolic and diastolic pressures are about 25 and 8 mm Hg, respectively (Fig. 1–10). By contrast, the mean pressure in the aorta is about 100 mm Hg. Since the pressures in the right and left atriums are not very dissimilar, about 2 and 5 mm Hg, respectively, the pressure differences from inlet to outlet of the pulmonary and systemic systems are about 10 (15 – 5) and 98 (100 – 2) mm Hg, respectively; that is, they differ by a factor of nearly 10.

In keeping with these low pressures, the walls of the pulmonary artery and its branches are remarkably thin, and they are easily mistaken for veins. This is in striking contrast to the systemic circulation where the arteries generally have thick walls, and the arterioles in particular have abundant smooth muscle.

The reasons for these differences become clear when the functions of the two circulations are compared. The systemic circulation regulates the supply of blood to various organs,

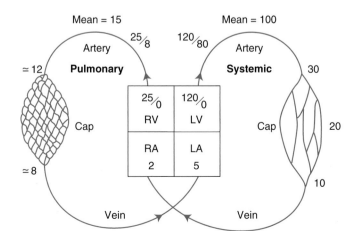

FIGURE 1–10. Comparison of pressures (mm Hg) in the pulmonary and systemic circulations at rest. Hydrostatic differences modify these. On exercise the pressures in the pulmonary circulation increase.

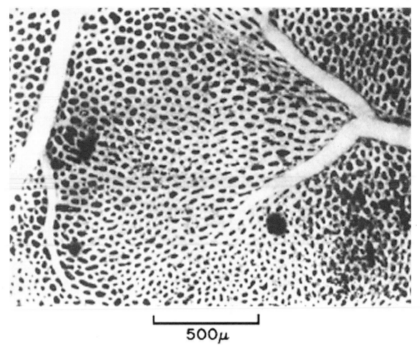

500μ

FIGURE 1–11. View of an alveolar wall (in a frog) showing the dense network of capillaries. A small artery (left) and vein (right) can also be seen. The individual capillary segments are so short that the blood forms an almost continuous sheet.

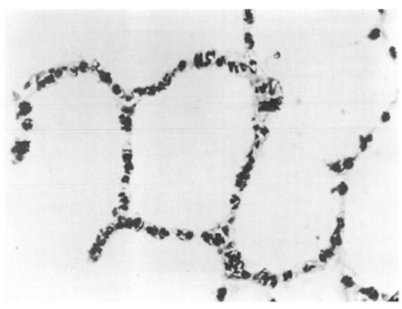

FIGURE 1–12. Thin microscopic section of a dog lung showing capillaries in the alveolar walls. The blood-gas barrier is so thin that it cannot be identified here (compare with Fig. 1–7).

including those which may be far above the level of the heart (the upstretched arm, for example). By contrast, the lung is required to accept the whole of the cardiac output at all times and is rarely concerned with directing blood from one region to another. Its arterial pressure is therefore as low as is consistent with lifting blood to the top of the lung.

The pressure inside the pulmonary capillaries is about halfway between pulmonary arterial and venous pressure, and probably much of the pressure drop occurs within the capillary bed itself (Fig. 1–10). This means that the distribution of pressures along the pulmonary circulation is far more symmetrical than in its systemic counterpart, where most of the pressure drop is just upstream of the capillaries (Fig. 1–10).

The pressure *around* the pulmonary capillaries is alveolar pressure, as would be expected from their structure as shown in Figure 1–7. Alveolar pressure is the same as atmospheric pressure when there is no flow through the airways. However, the pressure around the small pulmonary arteries and veins within the lung can be considerably less than alveolar pressure. As the lung expands, these "extra-alveolar vessels," as they are called, are pulled open by the radial traction of the elastic lung parenchyma which surround them **(FIGURE 1–13)**. Consequently, the effective pressure around these vessels is low and is comparable to the pressure around the

whole lung (intrapleural pressure). Both the small arteries and veins increase their caliber as the lung expands.

Cardiac Output

The whole of the output of the right heart goes through the lungs. Cardiac output at rest is 5 to 6 $l \cdot min^{-1}$ but can increase to approximately $25\ l \cdot min^{-1}$ during heavy exercise (Fig. 1–1B). Total pulmonary blood flow, and therefore cardiac output, can be measured using the Fick principle. This states that the O_2 consumption per minute ($\dot{V}_{O_2}$), measured at the mouth, is equal to the amount of O_2 taken up by the blood in the lungs per minute. Since the O_2 concentration in the blood entering the lungs is $C\bar{v}_{O_2}$ and that in the blood leaving the lungs is Ca_{O_2}, we have:

$$\dot{V}_{O_2} = \dot{Q}(Ca_{O_2} - C\bar{v}_{O_2})$$

or:

$$\dot{Q} = \frac{\dot{V}_{O_2}}{Ca_{O_2} - C\bar{v}_{O_2}}$$

$\dot{V}_{O_2}$ is measured by collecting the expired gas in a large spirometer and measuring its O_2 and CO_2 concentrations as we saw earlier in connection with Figure 1–1A. Mixed venous blood is taken via a catheter in the pulmonary artery, and arterial blood by puncture of a radial artery.

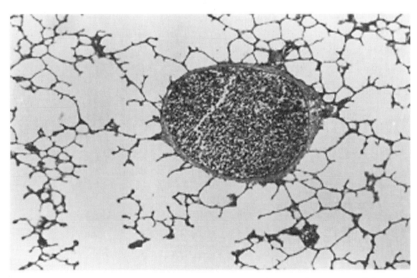

FIGURE 1–13. Section of lung showing many alveoli and an extra-alveolar vessel (in this case, a small vein) with its perivascular sheath. This vessel is pulled open by the radial traction of the surrounding alveolar walls.

Cardiac output can also be measured by indicator dilution techniques in which dye or another indicator is injected into the venous circulation and its concentration in arterial blood is recorded. These methods of measuring cardiac output are rather invasive, so in the case of Ann for the study shown in Figure 1–1B, a rebreathing method was used.

☐ CARRIAGE OF GASES BY THE BLOOD: HOW OXYGEN AND CARBON DIOXIDE ARE TRANSPORTED

Oxygen

We have seen that Ann is able to consume $3.5 \, l \cdot min^{-1}$ of oxygen when she is pedaling hard (Fig. 1–1A). How is the blood able to transport this large amount of oxygen to the peripheral tissues, chiefly the muscles of the legs? As just described, Ann's cardiac output at this high level of exercise is $25 \, l \cdot min^{-1}$ (Fig. 1–1B). Therefore, each liter of blood must be able to unload 3500/25 or 140 ml of oxygen per liter, that is $14 \, ml \cdot dl^{-1}$ of O_2. Furthermore, the blood traversing the muscle capillaries cannot afford to unload all its oxygen because it needs to maintain a certain partial pressure to ensure that oxygen diffuses to the mitochondria of the muscle cells in accordance with Fick's law (Fig. 1–8).

The challenge for the blood becomes clearer if we assume that oxygen can only be carried in the dissolved form. Oxygen obeys Henry's law, that is, the amount dissolved is proportional to the partial pressure (FIGURE 1–14). For each mm Hg of P_{O_2} there is $0.003 \, ml \cdot dl^{-1}$ of O_2 in the blood. Therefore, Ann's arterial blood, which has a P_{O_2} of about 100 mm Hg contains only $0.3 \, ml \cdot dl^{-1}$ of O_2 in the dissolved form. However, as we have seen, Ann's arterial blood needs at least $14 \, ml \cdot dl^{-1}$ of O_2. Therefore, the blood must contain a substance that can combine with large amounts of oxygen. As every high school biology student knows, this substance is hemoglobin.

Hemoglobin (Hb) is an iron-porphyrin compound joined to the protein globin, which consists of four polypeptide chains. The chains are of two types, α and β, and differences in their amino acid sequences give rise to various types of human Hb. Normal adult Hb is known as A. Hemoglobin F (fetal) makes up part of the Hb of the newborn infant. Hemoglobin S (sickle) has valine instead of glutamic acid in the β chains and this reduces its oxygen affinity. As a result, the dissociation curve is shifted to the right (see below) but, more importantly, the deoxygenated form is poorly soluble and tends to crystallize within the red cell. As a consequence, the cell shape changes from biconcave to crescent or sickle shaped, with increased fragility and a tendency to thrombus formation.

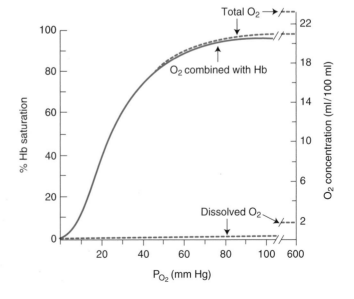

FIGURE 1–14. O_2 dissociation curve (*solid line*) for blood with pH 7.4, P_{CO_2} 40 mm Hg, and temperature 37°C. The total blood O_2 concentration is also shown for a hemoglobin concentration of $15 \, g \cdot dl^{-1}$ of blood.

Normal Hb A can have its ferrous iron oxidized to the ferric form by various drugs and chemicals including nitrites, sulfonamides, and acetanilid. This ferric form is known as methemoglobin. Another abnormal form is sulfhemoglobin. These compounds are not useful for O_2 carriage.

The *oxygen dissociation curve* describes the combination of Hb with oxygen (Fig. 1–14). Suppose we take a number of glass containers (tonometers), each containing a small volume of blood, and add gas with various concentrations of O_2. After allowing time for the gas and blood to reach equilibrium, we measure the P_{O_2} of the gas and the oxygen concentration of the blood. Knowing that 0.003 ml O_2 will be dissolved in each dl of blood per mm Hg P_{O_2}, we can calculate the O_2 combined with Hb (Fig. 1–14).

It can be seen that the amount of O_2 carried by Hb increases rapidly up to a P_{O_2} of about 50 mm Hg but above that the curve becomes flatter. The maximum amount of O_2 that can be combined with Hb is called the O_2 *capacity*. It can be measured by exposing the blood to a very high P_{O_2} (say, 600 mm Hg) and subtracting the dissolved O_2. One gram of pure Hb can combine with 1.39 ml O_2 and, since normal blood has about 15 $g \cdot dl^{-1}$ of Hb on the average, the O_2 capacity is about 20.8 $ml \cdot dl^{-1}$. Women tend to have lower Hb concentrations than men because of menstrual loss, and athletes also may have lower values because of an increased plasma volume. This explains Ann's value of 14 $g \cdot dl^{-1}$.

The *oxygen saturation of hemoglobin* is given by:

$$\frac{O_2 \text{ combined with Hb}}{O_2 \text{ capacity}} \times 100$$

The O_2 saturation with arterial blood with a P_{O_2} of 100 mm Hg is about 97.5%, while that of mixed venous blood with a P_{O_2} of 40 mm Hg (Fig. 1–9) is about 75%. The oxygen concentration of blood (in $ml \cdot dl^{-1}$) is given by:

$$\left(1.39 \times Hb \times \frac{Sat}{100}\right) + 0.003 P_{O_2}$$

where Hb is the Hb concentration in $g \cdot dl^{-1}$, Sat is the percentage saturation of the Hb, and P_{O_2} is in mm Hg.

The shape of the O_2 dissociation curve has several physiological advantages. The nearly flat upper portion means that even if the P_{O_2} in the blood falls somewhat, for example at high altitude (*see* Chapter 2), the O_2 concentration will be little affected. In addition, as the red cell takes up O_2 along Ann's pulmonary capillary (Fig. 1–9), a large partial pressure difference between alveolar gas and blood continues to exist even when most of the O_2 has been loaded. This helps the diffusion process (Fig. 1–8). The steep lower part of the dissociation curve means that Ann's exercising muscles can withdraw large amounts of O_2 for a relatively small drop in capillary P_{O_2}. This maintenance of blood P_{O_2} assists the diffusion of O_2 into the muscle cells. Because reduced Hb is purple, a low arterial O_2 saturation causes a blue coloration of the skin known as *cyanosis*.

The O_2 dissociation curve is shifted to the right (O_2 affinity of Hb is reduced) by increases in temperature, H^+ concentration, P_{CO_2}, and concentration of 2,3-diphosphoglycerate (2,3-DPG) in the red cell (**FIGURE 1–15**). Opposite changes shift the curve to the left. Most of the effect of P_{CO_2}, which is known as the *Bohr effect*, can be attributed to its action on H^+ concentration. A rightward shift means more unloading of O_2 at a given P_{O_2} in a tissue capillary. A simple way to remember these shifts is that Ann's exercising muscles are acid, hypercarbic, and hot, and they benefit from the increased unloading of O_2 from the capillaries.

2,3-DPG is an end product of red cell metabolism, and this shifts the curve to the right. An increase in concentration of this molecule occurs in chronic hypoxia, for example at high altitude, or in the presence of chronic lung disease. As a result, the unloading of O_2 to peripheral tissues is assisted. By contrast, stored blood in a blood bank may be depleted of 2,3-DPG and unloading of O_2 is therefore impaired. A useful measure of the position of the dissociation curve is the P_{O_2} for 50% O_2 saturation. This is known as the P_{50} and the normal value for human blood is about 27 mm Hg.

Carbon monoxide (CO) interferes with the O_2 transport of blood by combining with Hb to form carboxyhemoglobin (COHb). CO has about 240 times the affinity of O_2 for Hb; this means that CO will combine with the same amount of Hb as O_2 when the CO partial pressure is 240 times lower. The result is that small amounts of CO can tie up a large proportion of the Hb in the blood, thus making it unavailable for O_2 carriage. If this happens, the Hb concentration and P_{O_2} of blood may be normal but the O_2 concentration is greatly reduced. The presence of COHb also shifts the

O_2 dissociation curve to the left, thus interfering with the unloading of O_2. This is an additional feature of the toxicity of CO.

Carbon Dioxide

Just as Ann's tissues, chiefly her exercising muscles, are consuming $3.5 \text{ l} \cdot \text{min}^{-1}$ of O_2, so they are also producing about $3.5 \text{ l} \cdot \text{min}^{-1}$ of CO_2. This means that each dl of blood passing through her muscle capillaries has to load 14 ml of CO_2 so that this can be eliminated by the pulmonary capillaries. Actually, Ann's CO_2 output may even exceed $3.5 \text{ l} \cdot \text{min}^{-1}$ at maximal exercise because she may develop an unsteady state with a respiratory exchange ratio greater than 1.0. CO_2 is carried in the blood in three forms: dissolved, as bicarbonate, and in combination with proteins as carbamino compounds (**FIGURE 1–16**).

Dissolved CO_2, like O_2, obeys Henry's law, but CO_2 is some 20 times more soluble than O_2. The result is that dissolved CO_2 plays a significant role in its carriage in that about 10% of the gas that is evolved into the alveolar gas from the blood is in the dissolved form.

Bicarbonate is formed in blood by the following reactions:

$$CO_2 + H_2O \overset{CA}{\rightleftharpoons} H_2CO_3 \rightleftharpoons H^+ + HCO_3^-$$

The first reaction is very slow in plasma but fast within the red blood cell because of the presence there of the enzyme *carbonic anhydrase* (CA). The second reaction, ionic dissociation of carbonic acid, is fast without an enzyme. When the concentration of these ions rises within the red cell, HCO_3^- diffuses out, but H^+ cannot easily do this because the cell membrane is relatively impermeable to cations. Therefore to maintain electrical neutrality, Cl^- ions diffuse into the cell from the plasma, the so-called *chloride shift* (Fig. 1–16).

Some of the H^+ ions liberated are bound to Hb:

$$H^+ + HbO_2 \rightleftharpoons H^+ \cdot Hb + O_2$$

This occurs because reduced Hb is less acid (that is, a better proton acceptor) than the oxygenated form. Therefore the presence of reduced Hb in the peripheral blood helps with the loading of CO_2 while the oxygenation that occurs in the pulmonary capillary assists in the unloading.

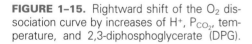

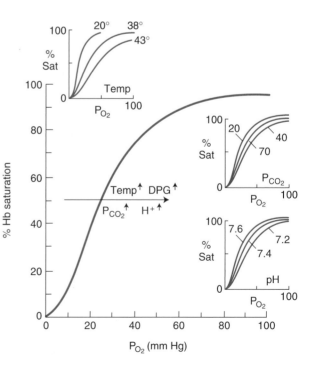

FIGURE 1–15. Rightward shift of the O_2 dissociation curve by increases of H^+, P_{CO_2}, temperature, and 2,3-diphosphoglycerate (DPG).

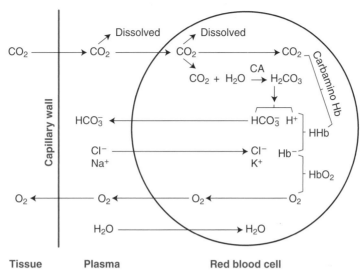

FIGURE 1–16. Scheme of the uptake of O_2 and liberation of CO_2 in systemic capillaries. Exactly opposite events occur in the pulmonary capillaries. See text for details.

The fact that deoxygenation of blood increases its ability to carry CO_2 is known as the *Haldane effect*.

Carbamino compounds are formed by the combination of CO_2 with terminal amine groups in blood proteins. The most important protein is the globin of Hb:

$$Hb \cdot NH_2 + CO_2 \rightleftharpoons Hb \cdot NH \cdot COOH,$$

giving carbamino-hemoglobin. Reduced Hb can bind more CO_2 as carbamino-hemoglobin than HbO_2. Therefore again, unloading of O_2 in peripheral capillaries facilitates the loading of CO_2, while oxygenation has the opposite effect.

Most of the CO_2 carried by the blood is in the form of bicarbonate with only small amounts as dissolved or as carbamino-hemoglobin. However, about 60% of the CO_2 that is loaded or unloaded by the blood comes from bicarbonate, 30% from carbamino-hemoglobin, and 10% from dissolved CO_2.

By analogy with the O_2 dissociation curve (Figs. 1–14 and 1–15), the relationships between CO_2 concentration and P_{CO_2} in blood can be referred to as the *CO_2 dissociation curve* (**FIGURE 1–17**). It can be seen that the dissociation curve for CO_2 is much more linear than that for O_2. In addition, the lower the saturation of Hb with O_2, the larger the CO_2 concentration for a given P_{CO_2}. This is a graphical representation of the Haldane effect referred to above.

□ BLOOD-TISSUE GAS EXCHANGE: HOW OXYGEN GETS TO THE TISSUE CELLS

O_2 and CO_2 move between the systemic capillary blood and the tissue cells by passive diffusion, just as they move between the capillary blood and alveolar gas in the lung. As Figure 1–8 shows, the rate of transfer of gas through a tissue sheet is proportional to the tissue area and the difference in partial pressure between the two sides, and inversely proportional to the thickness. The thickness of the blood-gas barrier is less than 0.3 μm in many places, but the distance between open capillaries in resting muscle is on the order of 50 μm. However, when Ann exercises hard, muscle blood flow increases and additional capillaries open up; this reduces the diffusion distance and increases the area for diffusion. Because CO_2 diffuses about 20 times faster than O_2 through tissue, elimination of CO_2 is less of a problem than O_2 delivery.

The way in which the P_{O_2} falls in tissue between adjacent open capillaries is shown schematically in **FIGURE 1–18**. As the O_2 diffuses away from the capillary, it is consumed by the tissue, and the P_{O_2} falls. In A, the balance between O_2 consumption and delivery (determined by the capillary P_{O_2} and the intercapillary distance) results in an adequate P_{O_2} in all the tissue. In B, the intercapillary distance or the O_2

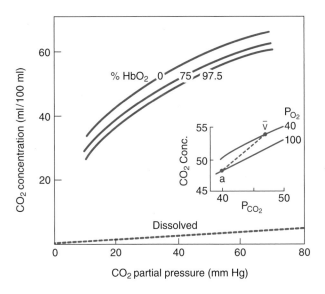

FIGURE 1–17. CO_2 dissociation curves for blood of different O_2 saturations. Note that oxygenated blood carries less CO_2 for the same P_{CO_2}. The *inset* shows the "physiological" curve between arterial and mixed venous blood as a *broken line*.

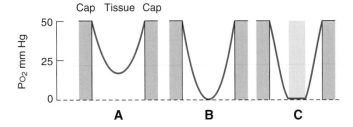

FIGURE 1–18. Diagram showing the fall of P_{O_2} between adjacent open capillaries in tissue. In **A**, oxygen delivery is adequate; in **B**, critical; and in **C**, inadequate for aerobic metabolism in the central core of tissue.

consumption has been increased until the P_{O_2} at one point in the tissue falls to zero. This is referred to as a *critical* situation. In C, there an anoxic region where aerobic (that is, O_2 utilizing) metabolism is impossible. Under these conditions, the tissue turns to anaerobic glycolysis with the formation of lactic acid.

There is recent evidence that much of the fall of P_{O_2} in some peripheral tissues occurs in the immediate vicinity of the capillary wall and that the P_{O_2} in the interior of muscle cells, for example, is very low (1 to 3 mm Hg) and nearly uniform. This pattern can be explained in part by the presence of myoglobin in the cell which acts as a reservoir for oxygen and facilitates its diffusion within the cell.

How low can the tissue P_{O_2} fall before O_2 utilization ceases? In measurements on suspensions of liver mitochondria in vitro, O_2 consumption continues at the same rate until the P_{O_2} falls to the vicinity of 3 mm Hg. Therefore, it appears that the purpose of the much higher P_{O_2} in capillary blood is to ensure an adequate pressure for diffusion of O_2 to the mitochondria and that at the actual sites of O_2 utilization the P_{O_2} may be very low.

Questions

For each question, choose the one best answer.
(For answers, see p. 150.)

1. **Maximal oxygen uptake ($\dot{V}_{O_2}$max):**
   A. Is the highest work rate that an individual can attain.
   B. Generally exceeds $6\,l \cdot min^{-1}$ in young, healthy females.
   C. Is the highest O_2 uptake attained when the work rate is incrementally increased.
   D. Is the O_2 uptake when the blood lactate suddenly rises during a test when the work rate is incrementally increased.
   E. Is the O_2 uptake when the total ventilation reaches a ceiling that cannot be exceeded.

2. **All of the following statements are true of inspiration during maximal exercise EXCEPT:**
   A. Diaphragm descends more than 3 cm.
   B. Lateral dimension of the chest increases.
   C. External intercostal muscles contract.
   D. Sternomastoid muscles contract.
   E. Intra-abdominal pressure falls.

3. **All of the following statements about the airways of the lung are true EXCEPT:**
   A. All the oxygen uptake occurs in the transitional and respiratory zones.
   B. Volume of the anatomic dead space is less than 10% of lung volume.
   C. Each acinus is supplied by a terminal bronchiole.
   D. The walls of the respiratory bronchioles are completely lined with alveoli.
   E. Alveolar ventilation is approximately equal to pulmonary blood flow under resting conditions.

4. **Two gases, A and B, have solubilities in tissue and molecular weights as follows:**

	Solubility	Molecular Weight
A)	24	36
B)	2	16

   If the two gases have the same partial pressure difference across a tissue sheet, the rate of diffusion of gas A through the sheet compared with the rate of diffusion of gas B is:
   A. 12:1
   B. 8:1
   C. 5.3:1
   D. 4:1
   E. 6:4

5. **All of the following statements are true about the blood-gas barrier in the human lung EXCEPT:**
   A. About half of the area of the barrier has a thickness of only 0.2 to 0.3 μm.
   B. The total area of the barrier is 50 to 100 m².
   C. The diffusion distance for O_2 across the thin side of the barrier is less than the average diffusion distance within the pulmonary capillary.
   D. The interstitium on the thick side of the blood-gas barrier is important for fluid exchange.
   E. Inflating the lung to high volumes can damage the blood-gas barrier.

6. **In a measurement of cardiac output, the O_2 concentrations in pulmonary arterial and systemic arterial blood were 16 and 21 ml · dl^{-1}, respectively, and the O_2 consumption measured at the mouth was 300 ml · min^{-1}. The cardiac output (in l · min^{-1}) was:**
   A. 3
   B. 5
   C. 6
   D. 12
   E. 60

7. **The presence of hemoglobin in normal arterial blood increases its O_2 concentration approximately how many times?**
   A. 10
   B. 20
   C. 40
   D. 70
   E. 100

8. **An increase in which of the following shifts the O_2 dissociation curve to the left?**
   A. Temperature
   B. P_{CO_2}
   C. H^+ concentration
   D. 2,3-DPG concentration
   E. Oxygen affinity of hemoglobin

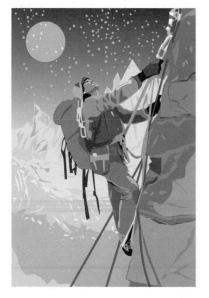

Chapter 2

Normal Physiology: Hypoxia

☐ Now we meet Bill, another medical student and an avid mountaineer. When Bill is exposed to the hypoxia of high altitude, he hyperventilates and this helps to maintain his alveolar P_{O_2}. We discuss how hyperventilation alters the oxygen cascade from the air to the tissues and how the fall in P_{CO_2} changes the acid-base status. Finally, we examine the mechanisms that regulate ventilation, including those that result in Bill's hyperventilation.

☐ ABOUT BILL

Meet Bill, another first-year medical student and an avid mountain climber. Bill is an excellent student, but outside his studies his great love is mountaineering. He began climbing seriously when he was in college and has now ascended a number of the highest peaks in the United States. Last year he made a trip to Argentina and successfully climbed Aconcagua (6960 m; 22,834 ft). His ambition is to climb Mt. Everest.

Bill is very aware of the debilitating effects of high altitude, including shortness of breath and difficulties with sleeping. He is also familiar with the advantages of acclimatization, and he has come across the illnesses associated with high altitude including acute mountain sickness, high-altitude pulmonary edema, and high-altitude cerebral edema. He is looking forward to understanding the scientific basis of these problems during his physiology course at medical school.

☐ BAROMETRIC PRESSURE AND ALTITUDE

Bill knows that the physiological problems at high altitude are caused by the low P_{O_2} in the air. This in turn is determined by the barometric pressure because at all altitudes of interest to us,

the composition of air is constant and contains 20.93% oxygen.

FIGURE 2–1 shows the fall in barometric pressure with increasing altitude. At an altitude of 5800 m (19,000 ft) the barometric pressure has fallen from its sea level value of 760 mm Hg to only about half that. At the summit of Mt. Everest the barometric pressure is only about 250 mm Hg, and at 19,200 m (63,000 ft) the barometric pressure is only 47 mm Hg.

How does this fall in barometric pressure affect the P_{O_2} of the inspired gas? As briefly mentioned in Chapter 1, when air is inhaled into the upper airways, it is warmed and moistened, and the water vapor pressure is then 47 mm Hg. This value depends only on the temperature of the body and essentially does not change in healthy people. This means that at sea level, the total dry gas pressure is $760 - 47 = 713$ mm Hg. The P_{O_2} of moist inspired gas is therefore $(20.93/100) \times 713 = 149$ mm Hg. We call the factor 20.93/100 the *fractional concentration* of oxygen, and its value in air is therefore 0.2093.

As we go to higher and higher altitudes, water vapor becomes increasingly important. On the summit of Mt. Everest the inspired P_{O_2} equals $0.2093 \times (250 - 47) = 42.5$ mm Hg. At an altitude of 19,200 m, the inspired P_{O_2} is $0.2093 \times (47 - 47) = 0$! In fact, at approximately

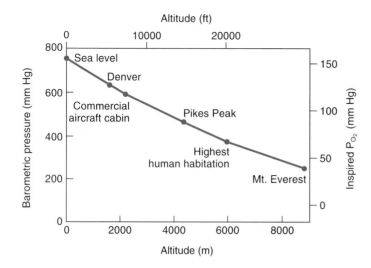

FIGURE 2–1. Relationship between barometric pressure and altitude. At 1580 m (5300 ft) (Denver) the P_{O_2} of moist inspired gas is about 130 mm Hg, but it is only 43 mm Hg on the summit of Mt. Everest.

this altitude, the tissues boil because their vapor pressure is equal to atmospheric pressure.

☐ OXYGEN CASCADE FROM AIR TO TISSUES

FIGURE 2–2 shows how the P_{O_2} in the body falls as oxygen moves from the atmosphere in which we live to the mitochondria where it is utilized. As we have seen, under normal conditions (solid line) the P_{O_2} of moist inspired air is $0.2093 \times (760 - 47)$ or 149 mm Hg (say 150). Figure 2–2 shows that by the time the O_2 has reached the alveoli, the P_{O_2} has fallen to about 100 mm Hg, that is, by one-third. This is because the P_{O_2} of the alveolar gas is determined by a balance between two processes: (1) the removal of O_2 by the pulmonary capillary blood, and (2) the continual replenishment of O_2 by alveolar ventilation. (Strictly, alveolar ventilation is not continuous but is breath-by-breath. However, the fluctuation of alveolar P_{O_2} with each breath is only about 3 mm Hg, so the process can be regarded as continuous.) The rate of removal of O_2 from the lung is governed by the O_2 consumption of the tissues and varies little under resting conditions. In practice, therefore, the alveolar P_{O_2} is largely determined by the level of alveolar ventilation. The same applies to the alveolar P_{CO_2} which is normally about 40 mm Hg.

In a hypothetical perfect lung, we can assume that the arterial blood has the same P_{O_2} as the alveolar gas because the P_{O_2} essentially equilibrates during the loading of oxygen in the pulmonary capillaries (*see* Fig. 1–9). When the arterial blood reaches the tissue capillaries, O_2 diffuses to the mitochondria where the P_{O_2} is much lower. The "tissue" P_{O_2} differs considerably throughout the body and, in some cells at least, the P_{O_2} is as low as 1 mm Hg. However, the lung is an essential link in the chain of O_2 transport, and any decrease of P_{O_2} in arterial blood must result in a lower tissue P_{O_2}, other things being equal. For the same reasons, impaired pulmonary gas exchange will also result in a rise in tissue P_{CO_2}.

Now, what happens to this scheme when Bill climbs to high altitude? Suppose he is at an altitude of 3185 m (10,500 ft) where the barometric pressure is only 525 mm Hg. The P_{O_2} of inspired gas is therefore $0.2093 \times (525 - 47) = 100$ mm Hg. If we assume that the difference between inspired and alveolar P_{O_2} remains at about 50 mm Hg, this gives an alveolar and arterial P_{O_2} of 50 mm Hg, and therefore a substantial fall in tissue P_{O_2} (*dotted line* in Fig. 2–2).

Can Bill do anything to mitigate this severe degree of arterial hypoxemia (abnormally low P_{O_2}) at high altitude? The answer is that he can (and does) by the process of hyperventilation. To understand this fully we have to become more quantitative. First, let's look at what determines the alveolar P_{CO_2} because this turns out to be simpler than the P_{O_2}.

FIGURE 2–2. Scheme of the fall of P_{O_2} from the inspired air to the tissues. The solid line shows the normal pattern at sea level. At an altitude of 3185 m (10,500 ft) the inspired P_{O_2} is only 100 mm Hg and, if alveolar ventilation is unchanged, the alveolar P_{O_2} will be only 50 mm Hg. However, hyperventilation raises the alveolar P_{O_2} to 75 mm Hg. The changes in tissue P_{O_2} reflect these changes.

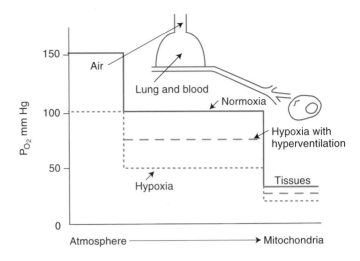

Hyperventilation

FIGURE 2–3 reminds us that the tidal volume (V_T) is a mixture of gas from the anatomic dead space (V_D) and a contribution from the alveolar gas (V_A) (compare with Fig. 1–6). However, since no gas exchange occurs in the anatomic dead space, and there is no CO_2 there at the end of inspiration, all the expired CO_2 comes from the alveoli.

Therefore:

$$\dot{V}_{CO_2} = \dot{V}_A \times \frac{\%CO_2}{100}$$

where $\dot{V}_{CO_2}$ is the CO_2 output and $\dot{V}_A$ is alveolar ventilation. As with the case of O_2 mentioned earlier, the term $\%CO_2/100$ is called the fractional concentration and is denoted by F_{CO_2}. Therefore, we can write the equation:

$$\dot{V}_{CO_2} = \dot{V}_A \times F_{CO_2}$$

Now the P_{CO_2} is proportional to the fractional concentration, or:

$$P_{CO_2} = F_{CO_2} \times K$$

where K is a constant and in this equation is simply the total dry gas pressure. Therefore,

$$\dot{V}_{CO_2} = \dot{V}_A \times \frac{P_{CO_2}}{K}$$

or:

$$P_{CO_2} = \frac{\dot{V}_{CO_2}}{\dot{V}_A} \times K$$

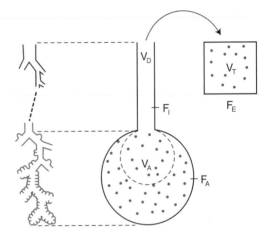

FIGURE 2–3. The gas in the tidal volume (V_T) is a mixture of gas from the anatomic dead space (V_D) and a contribution from the alveolar gas (V_A). The concentrations of CO_2 are shown by *dots* (compare with Figs. 1.5 and 1.6). *F*, fractional concentration; *I*, inspired; *E*, expired.

This is known as the *alveolar ventilation equation* and is remarkably simple. It states that the alveolar P_{CO_2} is inversely proportional to the alveolar ventilation if CO_2 production remains constant, as it generally does at rest. For example, if we double alveolar ventilation, alveolar P_{CO_2} will be halved from its normal value of 40 to 20 mm Hg.

Now we can go further and determine the relationship between the fall in alveolar P_{CO_2} and the rise in alveolar P_{O_2} that occurs with hyperventilation. To do this we use the *alveolar gas equation*:

$$P_{A_{O_2}} = P_{I_{O_2}} - \frac{P_{A_{CO_2}}}{R} + F$$

where R is the respiratory exchange ratio which is given by the CO_2 production/O_2 consumption and is determined by the metabolism of the tissues in a steady state, and F is a small correction factor (usually about 2 mm Hg during air breathing) which we can ignore. It is not necessary for us to derive this equation.

Let's use the alveolar gas equation to calculate Bill's alveolar P_{O_2} under various conditions. First, we have seen that at sea level the normal relationship between CO_2 production and alveolar ventilation gives an alveolar P_{CO_2} of 40 mm Hg. Therefore, assuming an inspired P_{O_2} of 150, a normal R value of 0.8, and ignoring F:

$$P_{A_{O_2}} = 150 - \frac{40}{0.8}$$
$$= 100 \text{ mm Hg}$$

This is the value shown by the solid line in Figure 2–2. Now suppose that Bill goes to high altitude where the $P_{I_{O_2}}$ is 100 mm Hg. If he does not change his alveolar ventilation or CO_2 production, his alveolar P_{CO_2} will remain at 40 mm Hg. The equation now gives:

$$P_{A_{O_2}} = 100 - \frac{40}{0.8}$$
$$= 50 \text{ mm Hg}$$

This is a severe degree of hypoxemia. However, if Bill doubles his alveolar ventilation (and his CO_2 production remains constant), his alveolar P_{CO_2} falls to 20 mm Hg, and the equation becomes:

$$P_{A_{O_2}} = 100 - \frac{20}{0.8}$$
$$= 75 \text{ mm Hg}$$

In other words, his alveolar P_{CO_2} has risen by 25 mm Hg. This procedure shows how powerful the process of hyperventilation can be in mitigating the effects of hypoxia of high altitude. In practice, Bill would have to go to a much higher altitude (actually about 6500 m or 21,300 ft) before his alveolar ventilation increased as much as twofold.

Figure 2–2 shows that under ideal conditions, the arterial blood has the same P_{O_2} as alveolar gas. In practice this is not quite attained, even in the normal lung, because while the capillary P_{O_2} continues to approach the alveolar value (*see* Fig. 1–9), it never quite gets there. In practice however, the difference is far too small to measure. However, failure of equilibration between the P_{O_2} of end-capillary blood and alveolar gas in the lung does occur under certain conditions. This was alluded to briefly in the discussion of Figure 1–9 (*see* Chapter 1). In fact, diffusion limitation of oxygen transfer across the blood-gas barrier frequently occurs at high altitude, particularly on exercise. Failure of diffusion equilibration also occurs when the barrier is thickened by disease. These topics are discussed further in Chapter 5.

There are two other reasons why the arterial P_{O_2} may be lower than the alveolar value. One is that, even in the normal lung, some blood finds its way into the arterial system without passing through ventilation regions of the lung. This mechanism is known as *shunt* and is discussed in Chapter 7, in which we shall see that this mechanism of hypoxemia can be of major importance in some types of disease. Secondly, mismatching of ventilation and blood flow in different regions of the lung results in depression of the arterial P_{O_2} below the mixed alveolar value. This difficult concept of ventilation-perfusion inequality will be discussed in Chapter 3.

☐ ACID-BASE STATUS

When Bill hyperventilated in response to the hypoxia of high altitude, and thus lowered his alveolar and arterial P_{CO_2}, important changes occurred in the acid-base status of his blood. To understand these, it is necessary to discuss the respiratory and metabolic aspects of acid-base regulation in general.

The pH resulting from the solution of CO_2 in blood and the consequent dissociation of carbonic acid is given by the Henderson-Hasselbalch equation. It is derived as follows. In the equation:

$$H_2CO_3 \rightleftharpoons H^+ + HCO_3^-$$

the law of the mass action gives the dissociation constant of carbonic acid K'_A as:

$$\frac{[H^+] \times [HCO_3^-]}{[H_2CO_3]}$$

Because the concentration of carbonic acid is proportional to the concentration of dissolved CO_2, we can change the constant and write:

$$K_A = \frac{[H^+] \times [HCO_3^-]}{[CO_2]}$$

Taking logarithms:

$$\log K_A = \log [H^+] + \log \frac{[HCO_3^-]}{[CO_2]}$$

whence:

$$-\log [H^+] = -\log K_A + \log \frac{[HCO_3^-]}{[CO_2]}$$

Since pH is the negative logarithm:

$$pH = pK_A + \log \frac{[HCO_3^-]}{[CO_2]}$$

Because CO_2 obeys Henry's law, the CO_2 concentration (mM) can be replaced by ($P_{CO_2} \times 0.030$). The equation then becomes:

$$pH = pK_A + \log \frac{[HCO_3^-]}{0.030\, P_{CO_2}}$$

The value of pK_A is 6.1, and the normal HCO_3^- concentration in arterial blood is 24 mM. Substituting gives:

$$pH = 6.1 + \log \frac{24}{0.030 \times 40}$$
$$= 6.1 + \log 20$$
$$= 6.1 + 1.3$$

Therefore,

$$pH = 7.4$$

As long as the ratio of bicarbonate concentration to ($P_{CO_2} \times 0.030$) remains equal to 20, the pH will remain at 7.4. The bicarbonate concentration is determined chiefly by the kidney, and the P_{CO_2} by the lung.

The relationships between pH, P_{CO_2}, and HCO_3^- are conveniently shown on a Davenport diagram (**FIGURE 2–4**). The two axes show [HCO_3^-] and pH, and lines of equal P_{CO_2} sweep across the diagram. Normal plasma is represented by point A. The line CAB shows the relationship between HCO_3^- and pH as carbonic acid is added to whole blood, that is, it is part of the titration curve for blood and is called the *buffer line*. The slope of this line is steeper than that observed for plasma separated from blood because of the presence of hemoglobin, which

has an additional buffering action. Also, the slope of the line measured on whole blood in vitro is usually a little different from that found in a patient because of the buffering action of the interstitial fluid and other body tissues.

The ratio of bicarbonate to P_{CO_2} can be disturbed in four ways; both P_{CO_2} and bicarbonate can be lowered or raised. Each of these four disturbances gives rise to a characteristic acid-base change.

Respiratory Alkalosis

This is the acid-base disturbance that occurs in Bill when he ascends to high altitude. As we have seen, there is a decrease in arterial P_{CO_2}, and this increases the HCO_3^-/P_{CO_2} ratio and thus elevates the pH (movement from A to C in Fig. 2–4). Whenever the P_{CO_2} falls, the bicarbonate concentration must also decrease to some extent because there is less carbonic acid in the blood. This is reflected by the right downward slope of the blood buffer line in Figure 2–4. However, the ratio HCO_3^-/P_{CO_2} rises. The hyperventilation accompanying exposure to high altitude is a good example of respiratory alkalosis, but other causes include hyperventilation caused by anxiety or overventilation by an anesthesiologist during surgery. As Figure 2–4 shows, an acute reduction of the P_{CO_2} from 40 to 20 mm Hg is associated with an increase in pH from 7.4 to about 7.6. A useful rule of thumb is that doubling or halving the P_{CO_2} causes a change in pH of about 0.2 units.

If Bill goes rapidly to a high enough altitude, the movement of his blood will correspond to moving from point A to point C in Figure 2–4. However, if he then remains at this altitude, the kidney will respond by increasing the elimination of bicarbonate in the urine. It is prompted to do this by the reduced P_{CO_2} in the renal tubular cells. The resulting reduction in plasma HCO_3^- then moves the HCO_3^-/P_{CO_2} ratio down toward its normal level. This corresponds to the movement from C to F along the line P_{CO_2} = 20 mm Hg in Figure 2–4B and is known as *compensated respiratory alkalosis*. Typical events would be:

$$pH = 6.1 + \log \frac{24}{0.030 \times 40} = 6.1 + \log 20 = 7.4 \quad \text{(Normal)}$$

$$pH = 6.1 + \log \frac{20}{0.030 \times 20} = 6.1 + \log 33.3 = 7.62$$

(Respiratory Alkalosis)

$$pH = 6.1 + \log \frac{13}{0.030 \times 20} = 6.1 + \log 21.7 = 7.44$$

(Compensated Respiratory Alkalosis)

A

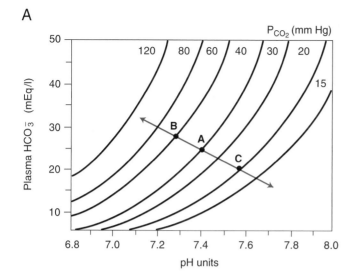

B

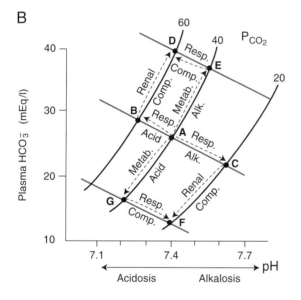

FIGURE 2–4. Davenport diagram showing the relationships between plasma bicarbonate concentration, pH, and P_{CO_2}. **A.** The normal blood buffer line BAC. **B.** The changes occurring in respiratory and metabolic alkalosis and acidosis (see text). The vertical distance between buffer lines such as BAC and DE, or GF, is called the *base excess*.

The renal compensation is usually not complete and so the pH does not fully return to its normal value of 7.4. The extent of the renal compensation can be determined from the *base excess*. This is the vertical distance between the two buffer lines. For full compensation, the buffer lines are AC and GF, and the vertical distance between them is about 13 mEq · l⁻¹. This is a negative base excess, sometimes called a *base deficit*. Because Bill did not have complete compensation of his respiratory alkalosis, the negative base excess or base deficit was a somewhat smaller number.

Respiratory Acidosis

This is caused by an increase in P_{CO_2}, and the subsequent events are exactly opposite to those for respiratory alkalosis. The HCO_3^-/P_{CO_2} ratio is reduced and this depresses the pH. This corresponds to a movement from A to B in Figure 2–4. An increase in P_{CO_2} is caused by hypoventilation, for example an overdose of a barbiturate, or ventilation-perfusion ratio inequality, as in chronic obstructive pulmonary disease (*see* Chapter 3).

If respiratory acidosis persists, the kidney responds by conserving bicarbonate. The resulting increase in plasma HCO_3^- then moves the HCO_3^-/P_{CO_2} ratio back up toward its normal level. This corresponds to the movement from B to D along the line $P_{CO_2} = 60$ mm Hg in Figure 2–4B. The result is *compensated respiratory acidosis*, but the compensation is rarely complete and so the pH does not fully return to its normal value of 7.4. Again, the extent of the renal compensation can be determined from the base excess, which is the vertical distance between the buffer lines BA and DE for full compensation.

Metabolic Acidosis

In this context, "metabolic" means a primary change in plasma bicarbonate, that is the numerator of the Henderson-Hasselbalch equation. In metabolic acidosis, the HCO_3^-/P_{CO_2} ratio falls, thus depressing the pH. The HCO_3^- may be lowered by the accumulation of acids in the blood, as in uncontrolled diabetes mellitus, or accompanying tissue hypoxia which releases lactic acid (*see* Fig. 1–1B). The corresponding change in Figure 2–4B is a movement from A toward G.

In this instance, respiratory compensation occurs by an increase in ventilation which lowers the P_{CO_2} and raises the depressed HCO_3^-/P_{CO_2} ratio. The stimulus to raise the ventilation is chiefly the action of H^+ ions on the peripheral chemoreceptors (see next section). In Figure 2–4B, the point moves in the direction of G to F (although not as far as F). There is a base deficit, or negative base excess.

Metabolic Alkalosis

Here an increase in plasma bicarbonate raises the HCO_3^-/P_{CO_2} ratio and, therefore, the pH. Excessive ingestion of alkalis, or loss of acid gastric secretion as in prolonged vomiting, are causes. In Figure 2–4B, the movement is in the direction A to E. Respiratory compensation sometimes occurs by a reduction in alveolar ventilation that raises the P_{CO_2}. Point E then moves in the direction of D (although never all the way). However, respiratory compensation in metabolic alkalosis is often small and may be absent altogether. Base excess is increased.

Mixed respiratory and metabolic disturbances often occur and may make it difficult to unravel the sequence of events.

☐ CONTROL OF VENTILATION

Principles

We have seen that when Bill ascends to high altitude, there is an increase in ventilation that reduces the alveolar P_{CO_2} and raises the alveolar P_{O_2}. This is clearly advantageous because it tends to maintain the arterial P_{O_2} in the face of the fall in the P_{O_2} of the air around Bill at high altitude. In fact, this process can be considered as a defense mechanism which, to some extent, protects the arterial P_{O_2} against the hypoxia of the environment.

What is the physiological mechanism that is responsible for raising Bill's ventilation? The answer to this question brings us to the topic of the control of ventilation. We will consider this in some detail here because it recurs again and again in our discussions of patients with lung disease.

The key role of alveolar ventilation in determining the alveolar (and therefore arterial) P_{CO_2} and P_{O_2} was discussed in relation to Figure 2–2. In this section we shall see that despite widely differing demands for O_2 uptake and CO_2 output made by the body, the arterial P_{CO_2} and P_{O_2} are normally kept within close limits. This remarkable regulation of gas exchange is possible because the level of ventilation is so carefully controlled.

The three basic elements of the respiratory control system (**FIGURE 2–5**) are as follows:

1. *Sensors* which gather information and feed it to the
2. *Central controller* in the brain which coordinates the information and, in turn, sends impulses to the
3. *Effectors* (respiratory muscles) which cause ventilation.

We shall see that increased activity of the effectors generally results in decreased sensory input to the brain, for example by decreasing the arterial P_{CO_2}. This is an example of negative feedback.

Central Controller

Brainstem

The periodic nature of inspiration and expiration is controlled by neurons located in the pons and medulla. These have been designated *respiratory centers*. However, they should not be

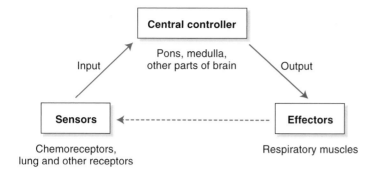

FIGURE 2–5. Three basic elements of the respiratory control system. Information from various sensors is fed to the central controller, the output of which goes to the respiratory muscles. By changing ventilation, the respiratory muscles reduce perturbations of these sensors (negative feedback).

thought of as comprising a discrete nucleus, but rather as a somewhat poorly defined collection of neurons with various components.

Three main groups of neurons are recognized.

1. *Medullary respiratory center* in the reticular formation of the medulla beneath the floor of the fourth ventricle. There are two identifiable areas. A group of cells in the dorsal region of the medulla (*dorsal respiratory group*) is chiefly associated with inspiration; another group in the ventral area (*ventral respiratory group*) is mainly for expiration. The cells in the dorsal respiratory group apparently have the property of intrinsic periodic firing, and they are responsible for the basic rhythm of ventilation. They generate repetitive bursts of action potentials when all known afferent stimuli to them have been abolished. Nervous impulses from these cells travel to the diaphragm and other inspiratory muscles.

The intrinsic rhythm pattern of the inspiratory area starts with a latent period of several seconds during which there is no activity. Action potentials then begin to appear, increasing in a crescendo over the next few seconds. During this time, inspiratory muscle activity becomes stronger in a "ramp"-type pattern. Finally, the inspiratory action potentials cease, and inspiratory muscle tone falls to its preinspiratory level.

The inspiratory ramp can be turned off prematurely by impulses from the *pneumotaxic center* (see below), which are inhibitory. In this way, inspiration is shortened and, as a consequence, breathing rate increases. The output of the inspiratory cells is further modulated by impulses from the vagal and glossopharyngeal nerves, which terminate in the tractus solitarius close to the inspiratory area.

The *expiratory area* is quiescent during normal breathing. However, as discussed in Chapter 1, expiration becomes active during exercise. This is the result of firing of the expiratory cells.

2. *Apneustic center* in the lower pons. This receives its name because if the brain of an experimental animal is sectioned just above this site, prolonged inspiratory gasps (apneuses) are seen. Its role in humans is unclear.

3. *Pneumotaxic center* in the upper pons. As indicated above, this area appears to "switch off" or inhibit inspiration and thus can regulate volume and rate. This center may be involved in fine-tuning respiratory rhythm.

Cortex

Breathing is under voluntary control to a considerable extent, and the cortex can override the function of the brainstem within limits. Voluntary hyperventilation is easy, and breath holding is possible within limits.

Other parts of the brain such as the limbic system and hypothalamus can alter the pattern of breathing.

Effectors

The muscles of respiration, particularly the diaphragm, were discussed in Chapter 1 (*see* Figs. 1–2 and 1–3).

Sensors

Central Chemoreceptors

A chemoreceptor is a receptor that responds to a change in the chemical composition of the blood or other fluid around it. The most important receptors involved in the minute-by-minute control of ventilation are those situated near the ventral surface of the medulla. In animals, local application of H^+ or dissolved CO_2 to this area stimulates breathing within a few seconds. At one time it was thought that the medullary respiratory center itself was the site of action of CO_2, but it is now accepted that the chemoreceptors are anatomically separate.

The central chemoreceptors are surrounded by brain extracellular fluid (ECF) and respond to changes in its H^+ concentration. An increase in H^+ concentration stimulates ventilation, whereas a decrease inhibits it. The composition of the ECF around the receptors is governed by the cerebral spinal fluid (CSF), local blood flow, and local metabolism.

Of these, the CSF is apparently the most important. It is separated from the blood by the blood-brain barrier (**FIGURE 2–6**), which is relatively impermeable to H^+ and HCO_3^- ions, although molecular CO_2 diffuses across it easily. When the blood P_{CO_2} rises, CO_2 diffuses into the CSF from the cerebral blood vessels, liberating H^+ ions which stimulate the chemoreceptors. Therefore the CO_2 level in blood regulates ventilation chiefly by its effect on the pH of the CSF. The resulting hyperventilation reduces the P_{CO_2} in the blood and therefore in the CSF. The cerebral vasodilatation that accompanies an increased arterial P_{CO_2} enhances diffusion of CO_2 into the CSF and the brain ECF.

The normal pH of the CSF is 7.32, and since the CSF contains much less protein than blood, it has a much lower buffering capacity. As a result, the change in CSF pH for a given change in P_{CO_2} is greater than in blood. If the CSF pH is displaced over a prolonged period, a compensatory change in HCO_3^- occurs as a result of transport of this ion across the blood-brain barrier. However, CSF pH does not usually return all the way to 7.32. The change in CSF pH occurs more promptly than the change of the pH of arterial blood by renal compensation (Fig. 2–4), a process that takes 2 to 3 days. Because CSF pH returns to near its normal value more rapidly than blood pH, CSF pH has a more important effect on changes in the level of ventilation and the level of the arterial P_{CO_2}.

Peripheral Chemoreceptors

These are the receptors that are responsible for Bill's increase in ventilation at high altitude. They are located in the carotid bodies at the bifurcation of the common carotid arteries and in the aortic bodies above and below the aortic arch. The carotid bodies are the most important in humans. They contain glomus cells of two types. Type I cells show an intense fluorescent staining because of their large content of dopamine. These cells are in close apposition to endings of the afferent carotid sinus nerve (**FIGURE 2–7A**). The carotid body also contains type II cells and a rich supply of capillaries. The precise mechanism of the carotid bodies is still uncertain, but it is generally believed that the glomus cells are the sites of chemoreception and that modulation of neurotransmitter release from the glomus cells by physiological and chemical stimuli affects the discharge rate of the carotid body afferent fibers (Fig. 2–7B).

The peripheral chemoreceptors respond to decreases in arterial P_{O_2} and pH as well as increases in arterial P_{CO_2}. They are unique among tissues of the body in that their sensitivity

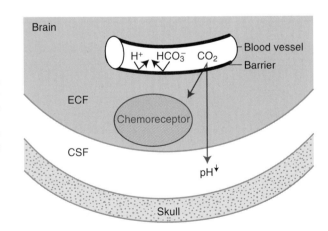

FIGURE 2–6. The central chemoreceptors are bathed in brain extracellular fluid (ECF) through which CO_2 easily diffuses from blood vessels to cerebrospinal fluid (CSF). The CO_2 reduces the CSF pH, thus stimulating the chemoreceptor. H^+ and HCO_3^- ions cannot easily cross the blood-brain barrier.

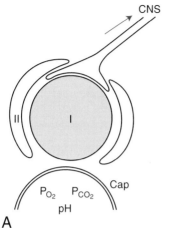

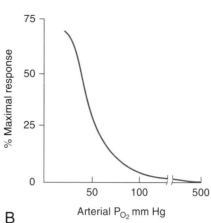

FIGURE 2–7. A. A carotid body which responds to changes of P_{O_2}, P_{CO_2}, and pH in arterial blood. *CNS*, central nervous system. **B.** The nonlinear response to arterial P_{O_2}. The maximal response occurs below a P_{O_2} of about 50 mm Hg.

to changes in arterial P_{O_2} begins around 500 mm Hg. Figure 2–7B shows that the relationship between firing rate and arterial P_{O_2} is very nonlinear. Some change occurs with an arterial P_{O_2} as high as 500 mm Hg but the response is much greater when the P_{O_2} falls below 70 mm Hg. The carotid bodies have a very high blood flow for their size; therefore, despite their high metabolic rate, the arterial-venous O_2 difference is small. As a result, they respond to arterial rather than venous P_{O_2}. The response of the receptors is very fast, and their discharge rate alters during the respiratory cycle as a result of the small cyclic changes in blood gases. The peripheral chemoreceptors are responsible for all of Bill's increase in ventilation in response to arterial hypoxemia. In fact, in the absence of these receptors, severe hypoxemia may depress respiration, presumably through a direct effect on the respiratory centers.

The response of the peripheral chemoreceptors to arterial P_{CO_2} is less important than that of the central chemoreceptors. For example, when a normal subject is given a CO_2 mixture to breathe, less than 20% of the ventilatory response can be attributed to the peripheral chemoreceptors. However, their response is more rapid and may be useful in matching ventilation to abrupt changes in P_{CO_2}.

The peripheral chemoreceptors also respond to a fall in arterial pH. This is the main mechanism responsible for the respiratory compensation in patients with metabolic acidosis as described in relation to Figure 2–4.

Lung Receptors

Pulmonary stretch receptors discharge in response to distension of the lung, and the impulses travel to the brain in the vagus nerve. The result is that they inhibit further inspiration and therefore slow respiratory frequency, a phenomenon known as the Hering-Breuer inflation reflex. This was one of the first pulmonary reflexes to be described but whether it is important in humans in unclear.

Irritant receptors are located in the airways and are stimulated by noxious gases, including cigarette smoke. The reflex effects include bronchoconstriction and increased ventilation (hyperpnea).

Juxtacapillary or J receptors are located in the alveolar walls close to the capillaries. They respond to engorgement of the capillaries, and may be important in the rapid, shallow breathing and dyspnea (sensation of difficulty in breathing) associated with interstitial lung disease and pulmonary edema (*see* Chapters 5 and 7). Impulses from the J receptors travel up the vagus nerves.

Other receptors. Irritant receptors exist in the nose, nasopharynx, larynx, and trachea, and stimulation causes sneezing, coughing, bronchoconstriction, and laryngeal spasm. Joint and muscle receptors may stimulate ventilation during exercise. Arterial baroreceptors in the aortic sinus can reflexly alter ventilation as a result of changes in blood pressure. Pain and temperature receptors can also affect ventilation.

Integrated Responses

Now that we have looked at the various units that make up the respiratory control system (Fig. 2–5), let's examine the overall responses of the system to changes in arterial P_{CO_2}, P_{O_2}, pH, and exercise.

Response to Carbon Dioxide

The most important factor in the control of ventilation under normal conditions is the P_{CO_2} of the arterial blood. The sensitivity of this control is remarkable. In the course of daily activity with periods of rest and exercise, the arterial P_{CO_2} is probably held to within 3 mm Hg. During sleep it may rise a little more.

The ventilatory response to CO_2 can be measured by having the subject inhale CO_2 mixtures or rebreathe from a bag so that the inspired P_{CO_2} gradually rises. Bill had his response measured by rebreathing from a bag that was pre-filled with 7% CO_2 and 93% O_2. As he rebreathed, metabolic CO_2 was added to the bag but the O_2 concentration remained high. The result was that the P_{CO_2} of the bag gas increased at the rate of about 4 mm Hg/min but the arterial P_{O_2} never fell low enough for it to stimulate ventilation. When Bill's ventilation was plotted against his alveolar P_{CO_2} (using the end-expired value as a measure of this), a straight line was obtained with a slope of $2\ l \cdot min^{-1} \cdot mm\ Hg\ P_{CO_2}^{-1}$.

FIGURE 2–8 shows the results of other experiments in which the inspired mixture was continually adjusted to maintain a different (but constant) alveolar P_{O_2}. It can be seen that with a normal P_{O_2}, the ventilation increased by about 2 to 3 $l \cdot min^{-1}$ for each 1 mm Hg rise in P_{CO_2}. Lowering the alveolar P_{O_2} produced two effects: a higher ventilation for a given P_{CO_2}, and a steepening of the slope of the line. There is considerable variation between subjects.

Another way of measuring respiratory drive is to record the inspiratory pressure during a brief period of airway occlusion. The subject breathes through a mouthpiece attached to a valve box, and the inspiratory port is provided with a shutter. This is closed during an expiration (the subject being unaware) so that the first part of the next inspiration is against an occluded airway. The shutter is opened after about 0.5 sec. The pressure generated during the first 0.1 sec of attempted inspiration (known as $P_{0.1}$) is taken as a measure of respiratory center output.

A reduction in arterial P_{CO_2} is very effective in reducing the stimulus to ventilation. For

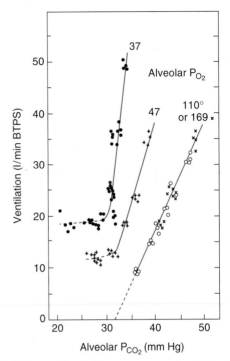

FIGURE 2–8. Ventilatory responses to CO_2. Each curve of total ventilation against alveolar P_{CO_2} is for a different alveolar P_{O_2}. In this study, no difference was found between an alveolar P_{O_2} of 100 mm Hg and one of 169 mm Hg, although some investigators have found that the slope of the line is slightly less at the higher P_{O_2}.

example, an anesthetized patient will frequently stop breathing for a minute or so if he or she is first overventilated by the anesthesiologist.

The ventilatory response to CO_2 is reduced by sleep, increasing age, and genetic, racial, and personality factors. Trained athletes and divers tend to have a low CO_2 sensitivity. Various drugs, including morphine and barbiturates, depress the respiratory center. Patients who have taken an overdose of one of these drugs often have significant hypoventilation. The ventilatory response to CO_2 is also reduced if the work of breathing is increased. This can be demonstrated by having normal subjects breathe through a narrow tube. The neural output of the respiratory center is not reduced, but it is not so effective in producing ventilation.

Response to Oxygen

Bill's ventilatory response to hypoxia was measured by having him rebreathe from a bag while he gradually consumed the O_2. During this time the end-tidal P_{CO_2} was held constant by absorbing some of the CO_2 in the bag. His arterial O_2 saturation was measured by a pulse oximeter which determines the color of the arterial blood in the finger. When the ventilation was plotted against arterial O_2 saturation, a straight line was obtained with a slope of $1.5\ l \cdot min^{-1} \cdot \%\ Sa_{O_2}^{-1}$, which is a normal value. Bill was relieved to find that he had a normal hypoxic ventilatory response because there is some evidence that climbers with a reduced response tolerate extreme altitude poorly—bad news if you hope to climb Mt. Everest some day!

FIGURE 2–9 shows the results of other studies of ventilatory response when the alveolar P_{O_2} was reduced and the alveolar P_{CO_2} was held constant at various values. It can be seen that when the alveolar P_{CO_2} was kept at about 36 mm Hg, the alveolar P_{O_2} could be reduced to about 50 mm Hg before any appreciable increase in ventilation occurred in these acute experiments. Raising the P_{CO_2} increased the ventilation at any P_{O_2} (compare with Fig. 2–8). When the P_{CO_2} was increased, a reduction in P_{O_2} below 100 mm Hg caused some stimulation of ventilation, unlike the situation when the P_{CO_2} was normal. Therefore, the combined effects of both stimuli exceeded the sum of each stimulus given separately; this is referred to as interaction between the high CO_2 and low O_2 stimuli.

Because the P_{O_2} can normally be reduced so far without evoking a ventilatory response, the role of this hypoxic stimulus in the day-to-day control of ventilation is small. However, as we have seen, when Bill ascends to high altitude, a large increase in ventilation occurs in response to hypoxia; this helps to maintain the alveolar P_{O_2} in the face of the low inspired P_{O_2} (Fig. 2–2).

Response to pH

A reduction in arterial blood pH stimulates ventilation. We saw earlier in this chapter that metabolic acidosis, as for example in uncontrolled diabetes mellitus, increases ventilation with the result that these patients have a low pH and low P_{CO_2} (Fig. 2–4B). The chief site of action of a reduced arterial pH is believed to be the peripheral chemoreceptors. However, it is possible that the central chemoreceptors are also affected by a reduction in blood pH if this is large enough. In this case, the blood-gas barrier apparently becomes partly permeable to H^+ ions.

Response to Exercise

We saw in Chapter 1 that Ann increased her ventilation enormously during severe exercise. Figure 1–1B (see Chapter 1) shows that her ventilation increased linearly with O_2 consumption up to a certain point, above which ventilation rose more rapidly, and this was associated with a large increase in lactate concentration in the blood. It is remarkable that the cause of the increased ventilation on exercise remains largely unknown.

Arterial P_{CO_2} does not increase during exercise; indeed during severe exercise (see right-hand part of Fig. 1–1B), it typically falls slightly because of the stimulation of ventilation by the lactic acid. The arterial P_{O_2} usually increases slightly, although it may fall at very high work levels in elite athletes because of diffusion limitation (see Fig. 1–9). The arterial pH remains nearly constant in moderate exercise, but in heavy exercise it falls because of the increase in blood lactate (see Fig. 1–1B). It is clear, therefore, that none of the mechanisms we have discussed so far can account for the large increase in ventilation observed in moderate exercise.

Other stimuli have been suggested. We referred earlier to joint and muscle receptors that may play a role. Another hypothesis is that oscillations in arterial P_{O_2} and P_{CO_2} with each tidal volume may stimulate ventilation even

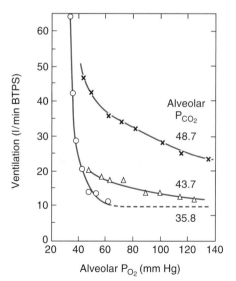

FIGURE 2–9. Ventilatory responses to hypoxia. When the P_{CO_2} is 36 mm Hg, almost no increase in ventilation occurs until the P_{O_2} is reduced to about 50 mm Hg.

though the mean levels remain the same. Another possibility is that the arterial P_{CO_2} chemostat (by analogy with a thermostat) is set to a lower level on exercise. Impulses from the motor cortex may be important, particularly in the early stages of exercise, and the increase in body temperature may play a role. However, none of the theories proposed so far is completely satisfactory.

☐ ACCLIMATIZATION AND HIGH-ALTITUDE DISEASES

High-Altitude Acclimatization

When a lowlander such as Bill goes to high altitude, a whole series of responses take place, a process known as acclimatization. This is one of the best examples of the way the human organism adapts to a hostile environment. The effectiveness of this process can be illustrated by pointing out that if Bill were acutely exposed to the barometric pressure at the summit of Mt. Everest (about 250 mm Hg) in a low-pressure chamber, he would probably lose consciousness within 1 or 2 minutes. However, many acclimatized mountaineers have now reached the summit of Mt. Everest without supplemental oxygen.

Hyperventilation

We have already seen that hyperventilation occurs at high altitude as a result of stimulation of the peripheral chemoreceptors by hypoxemia, and this has the effect of raising the alveolar and therefore arterial P_{O_2} (Fig. 2–2). This is the most important feature of acclimatization and indeed it is critically important at extreme altitude. As mentioned earlier, Bill's ambition is to climb Mt. Everest, and he hopes to do this without supplementary oxygen. However, as Figure 2–1 shows, the barometric pressure on the summit is only about 250 mm Hg, giving an inspired P_{O_2} of 43 mm Hg. Therefore, from the alveolar gas equation introduced earlier, if Bill maintained his normal alveolar ventilation, and therefore a P_{CO_2} of 40 mm Hg, and his respiratory exchange ratio was normal at 0.8, his alveolar P_{O_2} would be $43 - (40/0.8) = -7$ mm Hg! However, by increasing his alveolar ventilation fivefold and thus reducing his P_{CO_2} to 8 mm Hg, he can raise his alveolar P_{O_2} to $43 - 8 = 35$ mm Hg. This value just allows a small amount of physical activity. Of course, Mt. Everest is a very extreme

situation. Typically, the arterial P_{CO_2} in permanent residents at an altitude of 4600 m (15,000 ft) is about 33 mm Hg.

If Bill drives to an altitude of 3800 m (12,500 ft) in a day, his ventilation increases through hypoxic stimulation of his peripheral chemoreceptors. However, the resulting low arterial P_{CO_2} and alkalosis tend to inhibit this increase in ventilation. After a day or so, the CSF pH is brought partly back by movement of bicarbonate out of the CSF, and after 2 or 3 days, the pH of the arterial blood is returned to near normal by renal excretion of bicarbonate (Fig. 2–4B). These brakes on ventilation are then reduced, and it increases further. There is also evidence that the carotid bodies increase their sensitivity to hypoxia if this is sustained.

Persons born at high altitude tend to have a diminished ventilatory response to hypoxia that is only slowly corrected by subsequent residence at sea level. Conversely, those who are born at sea level and who move to high altitudes retain their hypoxic response intact for a long time. Apparently, therefore, this ventilatory response is determined early in life.

Polycythemia

Another feature of acclimatization to high altitude is an increase in the red blood cell concentration of the blood. The resulting rise in hemoglobin concentration, and therefore O_2 carrying capacity, means that although the arterial P_{O_2} and O_2 saturation are diminished, the O_2 concentration of the arterial blood may be normal or even above normal. For example, in permanent residents at an altitude of 4600 m (15,000 ft) in the Peruvian Andes, the arterial P_{O_2} is only 45 mm Hg, and the corresponding arterial O_2 saturation is only 81% (see Fig. 1–14). Ordinarily, this would considerably decrease the arterial O_2 concentration, but because of the polycythemia, the hemoglobin concentration is increased from 15 to 19.8 $g \cdot dl^{-1}$, giving an arterial O_2 concentration of 22.4 ml $\cdot dl^{-1}$, which is above the normal sea level value. The polycythemia also tends to maintain the P_{O_2} of mixed venous blood, and typically in Andean natives living at 4600 m, this P_{O_2} is only 7 mm Hg below normal (FIGURE 2–10).

The stimulus for the increased production of red blood cells is the low arterial P_{O_2} which causes hypoxia in some kidney cells. These release erythropoietin which in turn stimulates the bone marrow. As we shall see in Chapter 3,

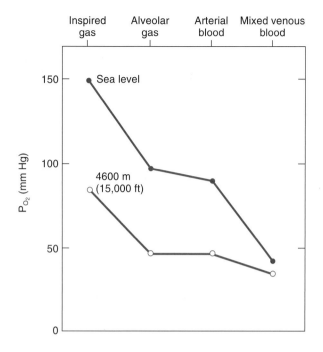

FIGURE 2–10. P_{O_2} values from inspired air to mixed venous blood at sea level and in permanent residents at an altitude of 4600 m (15,000 ft). Despite the much lower inspired P_{O_2} at the high altitude, the P_{O_2} of the mixed venous blood is only 7 mm Hg lower.

polycythemia is also seen in patients with chronic hypoxemia caused by lung disease.

Although polycythemia of high altitude increases the O_2 carrying capacity of the blood, it also raises the blood viscosity. This can be deleterious and some physiologists believe that the marked polycythemia that is sometimes seen at high altitude is an inappropriate response. For example, studies in the Peruvian Andes have shown that some permanent residents with severe polycythemia can increase their exercise ability if their red blood concentration is decreased by removing blood.

Other Features of Acclimatization

At moderate altitudes, there is a *rightward shift of the O_2 dissociation curve* (*see* Fig. 1–15) which results in better unloading of O_2 in venous blood at a given P_{O_2}. The cause of the shift is an increase in concentration of 2,3-diphosphoglycerate which develops partly because of respiratory alkalosis. However, the rightward shift interferes with the loading of O_2 in the lung. At extreme altitudes, a leftward shift occurs because of the marked respiratory alkalosis, and this is advantageous because it assists uptake of O_2 by the pulmonary capillaries. The *number of capillaries per unit volume* in skeletal muscle increases, mainly because the muscle

fibers become smaller. There are also changes in the *oxidative enzymes* inside the cells. However, the maximum O_2 uptake declines rapidly above 4600 m (15,000 ft).

Acute Mountain Sickness

Newcomers to high altitude frequently complain of headache, fatigue, dizziness, palpitations, insomnia, loss of appetite, and nausea. This is known as acute mountain sickness and is probably caused by a combination of hypoxemia and respiratory alkalosis. In most persons it disappears after 1 to 3 days.

Chronic Mountain Sickness

Long-term high-altitude residents sometimes develop an ill-defined syndrome characterized by cyanosis, fatigue, reduced exercise tolerance, marked polycythemia, and severe hypoxemia. This is called chronic mountain sickness and is best treated by descent if possible.

High-Altitude Pulmonary Edema

Lowlanders, such as Bill, who go to high altitude sometimes develop severe dyspnea, orthopnea (dyspnea is worse on lying down), cough, cyanosis, and rales (crackles) in the lung; this may progress to the point where they cough up pink, frothy fluid. This high-altitude pulmonary edema is life-threatening and should be treated by immediate descent. The mechanism is uncertain, but it is known to be associated with a high pulmonary artery pressure. When alveolar hypoxia occurs in a region of lung, there is local vasoconstriction of the small pulmonary arteries in that region. This is known as *hypoxic pulmonary vasoconstriction*, and is discussed in Chapter 6. At high altitude, where alveolar hypoxia occurs throughout the lung, pulmonary vascular resistance increases and therefore pulmonary artery pressure rises. How this causes pulmonary edema is uncertain, but one hypothesis is that the arteriolar vasoconstriction is uneven, and leakage occurs in unprotected, damaged capillaries. The edema fluid has a high protein concentration, indicating that the permeability of the capillaries is increased. Pulmonary edema is discussed in detail in Chapter 7.

High-Altitude Cerebral Edema

Lowlanders going to high altitude occasionally develop a condition characterized by confusion, ataxia (difficulty with walking), irrationality, hallucinations, and eventually clouding and loss of consciousness. Immediate descent is imperative. The mechanism is unclear, but the end result is leakage of fluid into the brain.

Questions

For each question, choose the one best answer.
(For answers, see p. 150.)

1. The P_{O_2} of moist inspired air (in mm Hg) at an altitude of 6500 m (barometric pressure 347 mm Hg) is:
   A. 53
   B. 63
   C. 73
   D. 83
   E. 93

2. A healthy medical student breathing air voluntarily hyperventilates and doubles his alveolar ventilation for several minutes. If his respiratory exchange ratio is 0.8 before and after the hyperventilation, approximately how much does his alveolar P_{O_2} rise in mm Hg?
   A. 20
   B. 25
   C. 30
   D. 35
   E. 40

3. If a climber on the summit of Mt. Everest (barometric pressure 247 mm Hg) maintains an alveolar P_{O_2} of 37 mm Hg and is in a steady state (R not greater than 1), his alveolar P_{CO_2} (in mm Hg) cannot be any higher than:
   A. 15
   B. 12
   C. 10
   D. 8
   E. 5

4. The laboratory provides the following report on arterial blood from a patient: pH 7.25, P_{CO_2} 32 mm Hg, and HCO_3^- concentration 25 mmol $\cdot$ l^{-1}. You conclude that there is:
   A. Respiratory alkalosis with metabolic compensation
   B. Acute respiratory acidosis
   C. Metabolic acidosis with respiratory compensation
   D. Metabolic alkalosis with respiratory compensation
   E. A laboratory error

5. A Hollywood socialite plans to climb Mt. Everest (barometric pressure 247 mm Hg) but wants to have the same P_{O_2} in moist inspired gas on the summit as at sea level. What does the O_2 concentration of the inspired gas (in %) need to be?
   A. 33
   B. 55
   C. 67
   D. 75
   E. 86

6. A patient with poliomyelitis and normal lungs is treated with mechanical ventilation, and CO_2 production remains constant. Without changing total ventilation, the arterial P_{CO_2} can be reduced by:
   A. Adding oxygen to the inspired gas
   B. Reducing the functional residual capacity
   C. Increasing the tidal volume
   D. Increasing the respiratory frequency
   E. Adding an external dead space

7. The arterial P_{CO_2} and bicarbonate concentration are both:
   A. Reduced in chronic respiratory acidosis
   B. Reduced in chronic metabolic alkalosis
   C. Elevated in chronic respiratory alkalosis
   D. Elevated in chronic metabolic acidosis
   E. Reduced by acute hyperventilation

8. All of the following statements about the brainstem and its role in ventilatory control are true EXCEPT:
   A. It contains neurons which generate the breathing rhythm.
   B. Its chemoreceptors are sensitive to changes in CSF pH.
   C. Its chemoreceptors are not directly sensitive to small changes in arterial pH.
   D. Its chemoreceptors are sensitive to changes in arterial P_{O_2}.
   E. It contains the tractus solitarius where impulses from the carotid chemoreceptors are received.

9. **All of the following statements about the peripheral chemoreceptors are true EXCEPT:**
   A. They respond to an increase in arterial blood pressure.
   B. They have a high blood flow per unit tissue mass.
   C. They respond to an increase in arterial P_{CO_2}.
   D. They respond to a decrease in arterial P_{O_2}.
   E. They respond to a fall in arterial pH.

10. **All of the following statements about the J (juxtacapillary) receptors are true EXCEPT:**
    A. They are located in the alveolar walls.
    B. They generate impulses that travel up the vagus nerve.
    C. They cause coughing when dust is inhaled.
    D. They may contribute to the rapid shallow breathing seen in pulmonary edema.
    E. They may contribute to dyspnea associated with interstitial lung disease.

11. **When a normal subject exercises by walking along the street, the ventilation increases because:**
    A. Arterial P_{CO_2} rises.
    B. Arterial P_{O_2} falls.
    C. Arterial pH falls.
    D. pH of the CSF falls.
    E. None of the above answers applies.

12. **Features of acclimatization to high altitude include all of the following EXCEPT:**
    A. Hyperventilation
    B. Polycythemia
    C. Rightward shift of the O_2 dissociation curve at extreme altitudes
    D. Increase in the number of capillaries per unit volume in skeletal muscle
    E. Changes in oxidative enzymes inside muscle cells

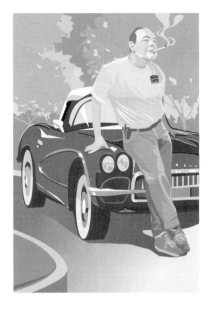

Chapter 3

Chronic Obstructive Pulmonary Disease

☐ Here we meet Chuck, a 60-year-old used-car salesman with severe chronic obstructive pulmonary disease, one of the commonest types of lung disease. First his clinical presentation is summarized, including his history, physical examination, laboratory investigations, and pulmonary function tests. We then see how the pathology and pathophysiology explain the findings. Topics covered include lung volumes, pressure-volume behavior of the lung, dynamic compression of the airways, and ventilation-perfusion inequality.

☐ CLINICAL FINDINGS*

History

Charles is a 60-year-old used-car salesman whose chief complaint is severe shortness of breath over the past 3 years. He was reasonably well until about 15 years ago when he began to notice that he had to pause to catch his breath after climbing a flight of stairs. Now he finds that he needs to stop for breath after walking about half a block on level ground. He has also had a chronic cough for about 15 years, and on several occasions each year, particularly in the winter, he has coughed up yellow, purulent sputum. He started smoking cigarettes when he was 15 years old, and for most of his life he has smoked two packs a day. During the past 12 months, he has noted intermittent swelling of his ankles associated with exacerbations of respiratory infections. There is no family history of lung disease.

As a used-car salesman, Charles is anxious to be on first-name terms with his prospective clients. His first request is, "Please call me Chuck," so we shall do this.

Physical Examination

The patient was dyspneic and somewhat florid in appearance with central cyanosis. Temperature was 38°C; blood pressure 150/80 mm Hg; pulse 80 beats · min^{-1}. There was slight neck vein engorgement. The chest appeared overinflated and barrel shaped. On auscultation of the chest with a stethoscope there was a generalized decrease in intensity of breath sounds. Occasional rhonchi (whistling sounds) were heard over both lungs. The liver was palpable one finger below the right rib margin. There was mild sacral and ankle edema.

Investigations

Hemoglobin concentration was 17 g · dl^{-1}. White blood cell count was 9500 · mm^{-3}. Sputum cultures failed to grow pathogens. A chest radiograph showed overinflation and abnormally

---

* The clinical findings are first briefly described here. Do not be concerned if you cannot understand all the details because they will be referred to again later in the chapter.

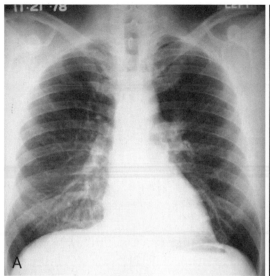
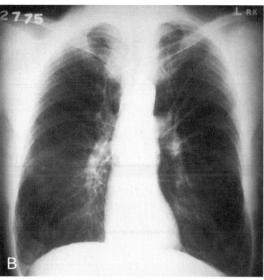

FIGURE 3–1. Chest radiographs. **A.** Normal appearance. **B.** Chuck's radiograph with the typical pattern of overinflation including low flat diaphragms, raised ribs, and a narrow mediastinum. There is also increased translucency of the lung fields. The original film showed attenuation and narrowing of peripheral pulmonary vessels, but these details do not reproduce well.

transradiant lung fields (**FIGURE 3–1**). An electrocardiogram (ECG) showed right axis deviation with tall P waves in lead 2. Right heart catheterization: mean pulmonary artery pressure was 30 mm Hg; pulmonary artery wedge pressure was normal.

Exercise Test

The patient walked on a treadmill in the pulmonary function laboratory. His maximal oxygen consumption was $1.2 \ l \cdot min^{-1}$.

Treatment and Progress

The patient was treated with bed rest, oxygen, bronchodilators, and diuretics, and gradually improved. He was advised to stop smoking and was able to comply. He also received subjective benefit from a rehabilitation program designed for patients with chronic lung disease, although this did not improve his $\dot{V}_{O_2}$max.

Subsequent History

The patient was admitted to the hospital 6 months later with an acute chest infection. His temperature was now 39°C, there was marked dyspnea with purulent sputum, cyanosis, rales (crackles) and rhonchi in all areas of the chest, and obvious ankle swelling. An arterial blood sample showed a P_{O_2} of 42 mm Hg, P_{CO_2} 55 mm Hg, and pH 7.30. The patient was treated with oxygen, antibiotics, bronchodilators, and diuretics. However, his condition worsened with increasing hypoxemia and a further increase in arterial P_{CO_2}. He died on the seventh day after admission.

Autopsy Findings

At autopsy the lungs were voluminous and failed to deflate normally. Some bronchi were filled with secretions. A large lung section showed many areas of parenchymal destruction (**FIGURE 3–2**). Histological examination revealed areas where the alveolar walls were destroyed (**FIGURE 3–3**). Some bronchial walls had enlarged mucous glands (**FIGURES 3–4 and 3–5**).

Diagnosis

Chronic bronchitis and emphysema leading to respiratory failure.

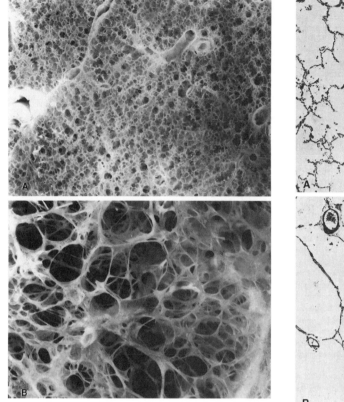

FIGURE 3–2. Appearance of slices of normal and emphysematous lung viewed with a hand lens. **A.** Normal. **B.** Severe emphysema with obvious breakdown of alveolar walls.

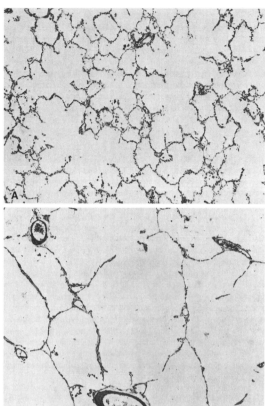

FIGURE 3–3. Microscopic appearance of emphysematous lung. **A.** Normal lung. **B.** Loss of alveolar walls with consequent enlargement of air spaces and loss of radial traction on small airways and blood vessels.

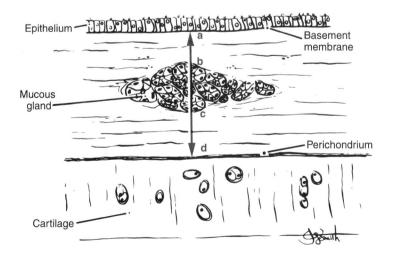

FIGURE 3–4. Diagram of the structure of a normal bronchial wall. In chronic bronchitis, the thickness of the mucous glands increases (*see* Fig. 3–5B). The thickness can be expressed as the Reid index given by (*b-c*)/(*a-d*).

☐ PATHOLOGY

Chuck showed many of the common features of chronic obstructive pulmonary disease, and we can learn much by discussing his clinical findings, laboratory investigations, pathology, and pathophysiology. Let's start with the structure of the lungs because many aspects of disordered function flow naturally from this.

Figure 3–2A shows the appearance of a slice of normal human lung fixed in the expanded state as seen with a hand lens. Small airways are clearly visible (compare with Figs. 1–4 and 1–5) and these lead into the alveolar region of the lung, often called the *parenchyma*. In Figure 3–2A, the alveoli look generally uniform throughout the section. By contrast, in Figure 3–2B which is at the same magnification, the normal lung structure has clearly been grossly disturbed, and large holes are visible where there should be fine alveolar tissue.

Additional information is given by microscopic sections of the lung as shown in Figure 3–3. Figure 3–3A shows normal lung, and the alveoli are clearly seen (compare with Fig. 1–12). The larger air spaces here are alveolar ducts (*see* Fig. 1–5). By contrast, in Figure 3–3B we can see that large numbers of alveolar walls have been destroyed, leaving large air spaces.

The appearances shown in Figures 3–2 and 3–3 are typical of the disease *emphysema*. A useful definition of this disease is that it is *characterized by enlargement of the air spaces distal to the terminal bronchiole (see Fig. 1–5) with destruction of their walls*. Strictly speaking, emphysema is an anatomical definition, and we rarely have the opportunity of seeing lung tissue from a living patient.

We can make some predictions about the functional abnormalities of the emphysematous lung by looking at Figures 3–2 and 3–3. Because the normal architecture of the lung has been destroyed, we might guess that its elastic behavior has been altered, and that lung volumes are abnormal. We might further expect that the resistance of the airways is increased because these are not held open by the radial traction of the surrounding parenchyma (compare with the blood vessel in Fig. 1–13). We might also predict that the resistance to blood flow through the lung is increased because many of the alveolar walls have been destroyed with the consequent loss of many pulmonary capillaries.

Figure 3–4 is a drawing of the normal structure of a bronchial wall showing the epithe-

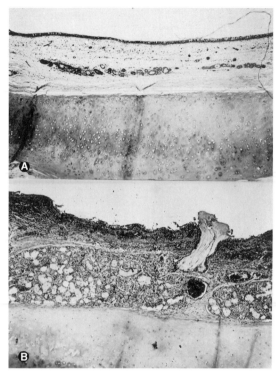

FIGURE 3–5. Histological changes in chronic bronchitis. **A.** Normal bronchial wall. **B.** Bronchial wall of Chuck's lung showing severe chronic bronchitis. Note the great hypertrophy of the mucous glands and the cellular infiltration.

lium, a subepithelial mucous gland, and cartilage. This will help us to identify the structures seen in the normal histological section of Figure 3–5A. By contrast, Figure 3–5B shows gross hypertrophy of the mucous glands in the airway wall. (The appearances may be confusing at first until we realize that essentially all the bronchial wall between the epithelium and the cartilage is occupied by the hypertrophied mucous glands.) As we shall subsequently see, these glands are responsible for producing the mucus that lines the airways, and they have hypertrophied in response to many years of insults from the inhaled tobacco smoke. The chronic inflammatory response has caused swelling of the bronchial walls, and some of the airways will be blocked by the excessive secretions. This condition is known as chronic bronchitis, and the disease is *characterized by excessive mucus production in the bronchial tree, sufficient to cause excessive expectoration of sputum.*

☐ PHYSIOLOGY AND PATHOPHYSIOLOGY

Armed with this knowledge of the anatomical pathology of this patient's lungs, we can now discuss the functional abnormalities that resulted in his clinical presentation, laboratory investigations, and subsequent history.

Clinical Presentation

The patient's chief complaint was increasing shortness of breath, and we can already see some reasons for this. His chronic bronchitis resulted in thickening of the bronchial walls and obstruction of some of them with secretions. His emphysema left many of his airways poorly supported and liable to collapse. However, a full analysis of why airway function was so abnormal must wait until later in this chapter. Chuck's complaint of ankle swelling will be considered in the next section.

Physical Examination

"Florid in appearance with central cyanosis." The suffused dark red coloration of his skin suggests an abnormally high hemoglobin concentration, and this was confirmed by the laboratory investigation showing that this was 17 rather than the normal 15 $g \cdot dl^{-1}$. The central cyanosis (bluish coloring of the conjunctivae of the eyes and mucous membranes of the mouth) suggests that the blood had an abnormally low oxygen saturation (see Fig. 1–14). This fits with the abnormally low arterial P_{O_2} of 58 mm Hg shown in TABLE 3–1. The low arterial P_{O_2} caused tissue hypoxia and, in the kidney, this resulted in the release of erythropoietin that stimulated the bone marrow to produce more red blood cells.

The appearance of overinflation of the chest suggests that lung volume was increased, and this was confirmed by the measurements shown in Table 3–1 which will be discussed shortly. The reduced intensity of the breath sounds is a common finding in patients with large lung volumes because these sounds are poorly transmitted to the chest wall. An additional factor may be the destruction of alveolar tissue shown in Figures 3–2B and 3–3B. The fact that whistling sounds were heard over both lungs is consistent with narrowing of some of the airways as a result of bronchitis, causing local turbulence and the generation of sounds. Airflow in the lung is considered in more detail in Chapter 4.

The neck vein engorgement, ankle edema (referred to both in the history and physical examination), and the palpable and therefore enlarged liver form a triad which is consistent

---

TABLE 3–1
Pulmonary Function Tests

Lung Volumes and Compliance	Observed	Predicted
VC (liters)	3.3	4.8
FRC (liters) by helium dilution	6.0	3.7
FRC (liters) by body plethysmograph	6.5	3.7
TLC (liters) by body plethysmograph	8.1	7.1
Compliance ($l \cdot cm\ H_2O^{-1}$)	0.35	0.20
Forced Expiration		
FEV_1 (liters)	1.3	3.6
FVC (liters)	3.1	4.8
FEV/FVC%	42	75
$FEF_{25-75\%}$ ($l \cdot sec^{-1}$)	1.4	3.6
Arterial Blood Gases		
P_{O_2} (mm Hg)	58	85
P_{CO_2} (mm Hg)	49	40
pH	7.36	7.40

with right heart disease. As was noted earlier, the destruction of many of the pulmonary capillaries means that the resistance to the flow of blood through the lungs (pulmonary vascular resistance) was increased. This is the reason why the pulmonary artery pressure was raised (see Investigations below) and also explains the changes in the electrocardiogram. Because the right heart is pumping against an increased pressure over a long period, the filling pressure of the right heart is increased, leading to neck vein engorgement, an enlarged liver, and dependent edema. The neck veins can be thought of as manometers measuring the pressure in the great veins. The presence of edema is explained by disturbance of the Starling equilibrium regulating the movement of fluid across the systemic capillaries, and this will be discussed in detail in Chapter 7.

Investigations

The white blood cell count of $9500 \cdot mm^{-3}$ was marginally raised, consistent with the low grade infection of the bronchi. The fact that sputum cultures failed to grow pathogenic organisms is common in these patients and is at least partly due to the fact that the patient was probably given some antibiotics.

Figure 3–1 contrasts the patient's chest radiograph with that of a normal subject. The patient's lungs are overinflated, as evidenced by the low flat diaphragms, elevation of the ribs, and narrow mediastinum. This indicates an abnormally large lung volume, and this is confirmed by the pulmonary function tests that will be considered next. The original radiograph showed abnormally dark lung fields, indicating that the lung tissue absorbed less of the X-rays than a normal lung. This is not surprising in view of the structure of the patient's lung, shown in Figures 3–2B and 3–3B. The destruction of much of the alveolar tissue means that the lungs did not absorb the X-rays as much as a normal lung.

The details of the ECG need not concern us here, but the right axis deviation is consistent with hypertrophy of the right heart, which goes along with the abnormally high pulmonary artery pressure of 30 mm Hg (compare with Fig. 1–10). The tall P waves in lead 2 are consistent with an enlarged right atrium caused by the high filling pressures for the right heart. It should be noted that cardiac catheterization is rarely indicated in this type of patient, and it is not clear

why this was done. However, it does allow us to document the pulmonary hypertension. The pulmonary artery wedge pressure, which is measured by wedging the catheter into a small pulmonary artery, is a measure of pulmonary venous pressure, and this is normal indicating that there is no failure of the left side of the heart.

Pulmonary Function Tests

The results of these are shown in Table 3–1 and will be discussed in some detail. First let's look at the *lung volumes*. Some of these can be measured with a spirometer (**FIGURE 3–6**). During exhalation, the lightweight bell goes up and the pen goes down, marking a moving chart. First, normal breathing can be seen (*see tidal volume* in Fig. 1–6). Next, the normal subject took a maximal inspiration and followed this by a maximal expiration. The expired volume is called the *vital capacity*. However, some gas remained in the lung after the maximal expiration; this is the *residual volume*. The volume of gas in the lung after a normal expiration is the *functional residual capacity*.

Neither the functional residual capacity nor the residual volume can be measured with a simple spirometer. However, a gas dilution technique can be used as shown in **FIGURE 3–7**. The subject is connected to a spirometer containing a known concentration of helium which is almost insoluble in blood. After some breaths, the helium concentrations in the spirometer and lung become the same. Since no helium has been lost, the amount of helium present before equilibration (concentration × volume) is $C_1 \times V_1$ and equals the amount after equilibration $C_2 \times (V_1 + V_2)$. From this, $V_2 = V_1 (C_1 - C_2)/C_2$. In practice, O_2 is added to the spirometer during equilibration to make up for that consumed by the subject, and also the CO_2 produced by the subject is absorbed.

Another way of measuring the functional residual capacity (FRC) is to use a body plethysmograph (**FIGURE 3–8**). This is a large airtight box, like an old telephone booth, in which the patient sits. At the end of a normal expiration, a shutter closes the mouthpiece and the patient is asked to make respiratory efforts. As he tries to inhale, he expands the gas in his lungs slightly, lung volume increases, and therefore the box pressure rises since its volume is decreased. Boyle's law states that pressure × volume is constant (at constant temperature). Therefore,

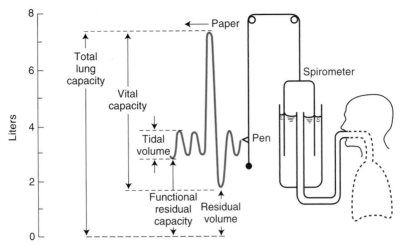

FIGURE 3–6. Lung volumes. Total lung capacity, functional residual capacity, and residual volume cannot be measured with the spirometer.

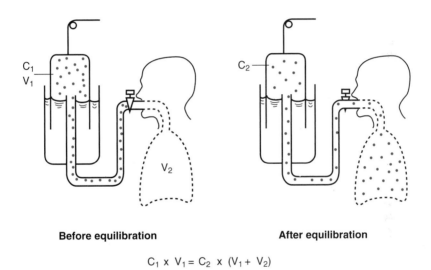

Before equilibration   **After equilibration**

$$C_1 \times V_1 = C_2 \times (V_1 + V_2)$$

FIGURE 3–7. Measurement of the functional residual capacity (V_2) by helium dilution.

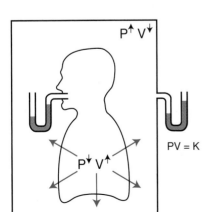

FIGURE 3–8. Measurement of FRC with the body plethysmograph. When a patient makes an inspiratory effort against a closed airway, he or she slightly increases the volume of the lung, airway pressure decreases, and box pressure increases. From Boyle's law, lung volume is obtained (see text).

knowing the pressures in the box before and after the inspiratory effort, and the preinspiratory box volume, we can calculate the change in volume in the lungs. Next, Boyle's law is applied to the gas in the lung. Since we know the pressures before and after the inspiratory effort, and the change in volume of the lung (which is the same as the change in volume of the box), the preinspiratory volume which is FRC can be derived.

Table 3–1 shows that Chuck's FRC was measured by these techniques, and that while the helium method gave a volume of 6.0 liters, the plethysmograph gave 6.5 liters. What is the reason for the difference? The body plethysmograph measures the total volume of gas in the lung, including any that is trapped behind closed airways and that therefore does not communicate with the mouth. By contrast, the helium dilution method measures only communicating gas, or lung that is ventilated in the time allowed for equilibration. In young normal subjects these volumes are virtually the same. However, in patients like Chuck there may be gas trapped behind obstructed airways, and there are certainly regions of the lung that are so poorly ventilated that they do not equilibrate. Therefore the helium volume is less than the plethysmograph volume.

Table 3–1 also shows that the FRC and total lung capacity (TLC) of Chuck were considerably higher than the predicted values of men of his age and height. To understand the reasons for this we need to look at the elastic properties of the lung.

Pressure-Volume Curve

Suppose we take an excised animal (or human) lung, cannulate the trachea, and place it inside a jar (**FIGURE 3–9**). When the pressure inside the jar is reduced below atmospheric pressure, the lung expands and its change in volume can be measured with a spirometer. The pressure is held at each level, as indicated by the points, for a few seconds to allow the lung to come to rest. In this way, a pressure-volume curve of the lung can be plotted.

In Figure 3–9, the expanding pressure around the lung is generated by a pump, but in humans it is developed by an increase in volume of the chest (*see* Figs. 1–2 and 1–3). The fact that the intrapleural space between the lung and chest wall is much smaller than between the lung and the bottle in Figure 3–9 makes no essential difference. The intrapleural space normally contains only a few milliliters of fluid.

Figure 3–9 shows that the curves that the lung follows during inflation and deflation are different. This behavior is known as *hysteresis*. Note that the lung volume at any given pressure during deflation is larger than during inflation. Also, the lung without any expanding pressure has some air inside it. In fact, even if the pressure around the lung is raised above atmospheric pressure, little further air is lost because small airways close, trapping gas in the alveoli. This *airway closure* occurs at higher lung volumes with increasing age and also in some types of lung disease, especially chronic obstructive pulmonary disease (COPD), as Chuck had.

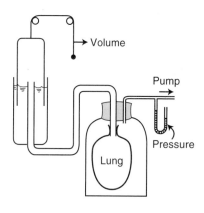

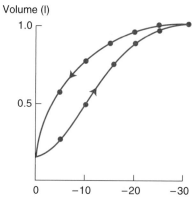

FIGURE 3–9. Measurement of the pressure-volume curve of excised lung. The lung is held at each pressure for a few seconds while its volume is measured. The curve is nonlinear and becomes flatter at higher expanding pressures. The inflation and deflation curves are not the same; this is called hysteresis.

In Figure 3–9, the pressure inside the airways and alveoli of the lung is the same as atmospheric pressure, which is zero on the horizontal axis. (The pressure in the spirometer bell is atmospheric.) Therefore this axis also measures the difference in pressure between the inside and outside of the lung. This is known as the *transpulmonary pressure* and is numerically equal to the pressure around the lung when the alveolar pressure is atmospheric. It is also possible to measure the pressure-volume of the lung shown in Figure 3–9 by inflating it with positive pressure and leaving the pleural surface exposed to the atmosphere. In this case, the horizontal axis could be labeled "airway pressure," and the values would be positive. The curves would be identical to those shown in Figure 3–9.

The slope of the pressure-volume curve, or the volume change per unit pressure change, is known as the *compliance*. In the normal working range (intrapleural pressure of about −5 to −10 cm water) the lung is remarkably distensible or very compliant. The compliance of the total human lung (both left and right lungs together) is about 200 ml · cm^{-1} water. However, at higher expanding pressures, the lung becomes stiffer, and its compliance is smaller, as shown by the flatter slope of the curve.

It is possible to measure a pressure-volume curve, such as that shown in Figure 3–9, in a living patient such as Chuck. In this case, the pressure around the lung is measured by means of a catheter inserted through the nose into the esophagus. Changes in esophageal pressure reflect changes in the pressure around the lung (intrapleural pressure) reasonably accurately. Typically, the patient is asked to breath in to TLC and then exhale in a series of volume steps while the pressure is measured. Normally, only the deflation limb of the pressure-volume curve is recorded. The slope is generally measured over the working range of the lung, for example 1 liter above FRC. Table 3–1 shows that for Chuck, the lung compliance measured in this way was 0.35 l · cm H_2O^{-1}, which was substantially higher than the predicted value of 0.20.

The compliance of the lung is increased in emphysema because the destruction of the normal architecture of the lung (Figs. 3–2B and 3–3B) means that the normal elastic recoil is reduced. The compliance also increases somewhat with age, possibly because of changes in the elastic tissue of the lung. The compliance is reduced by diseases that cause fibrosis of the lung, as we shall see in Chapter 5.

The normal elastic behavior of the lung depends in part on the fibers of collagen and elastin that can be seen in the alveolar walls and around the blood vessels and bronchi. When the lung is inflated, these fibers are stretched or, more probably, distorted, so they have a tendency to return to their original shape and therefore develop elastic recoil. However, in addition to these solid structures, the surface tension of the alveolar lining layer plays an important part in the elastic behavior of the lung, and this will be considered in Chapter 7. There is no evidence that abnormalities of surface tension play a part in the increased compliance of Chuck's lung. Here, the destruction of the normal architecture is the important factor.

We have seen that the increase in lung volume, for example FRC, in Chuck is due to the reduced elastic recoil of the lung. Strictly, the volume of the lung depends on a balance between the inward recoil of the lung and the outward recoil of the chest wall. The latter is presumably normal in Chuck (at least in the early stages of the disease). The interactions between the lung and chest wall will be considered more in Chapter 5.

Regional Differences of Ventilation in the Lung

So far we have tacitly assumed that all regions of the normal lung have the same ventilation. However, it has been shown that the lower regions of the lung ventilate better than the upper zones. This can be demonstrated if a subject inhales radioactive xenon gas (**FIGURE 3–10**). When the xenon-133 enters the counting field, its radiation penetrates the chest wall and can be recorded by a bank of counters, or a radiation camera. In this way, the volume of the inhaled xenon going to various regions of the lung can be determined.

Figure 3–10 shows that in the normal lung, the ventilation per unit volume is greatest near the bottom of the lung and becomes progressively smaller toward the top. Other measurements show that when the subject is in the supine position, this difference disappears, with the result that the apical and basal ventilations become the same. However, in that posture, the ventilation of the lowermost (posterior) lung exceeds that of the uppermost (anterior) lung.

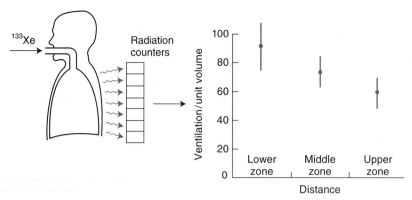

FIGURE 3–10. Demonstration of the regional differences in ventilation using radioactive xenon. When the gas is inhaled, its radiation can be detected by counters outside the chest. The ventilation decreases from the lower to upper regions of the upright lung.

Again, in the lateral position (subject on the side) the dependent lung is best ventilated.

An explanation for these topographical differences is shown in **FIGURE 3–11**. It is now known that the intrapleural pressure is less negative at the bottom than the top of the lung. The reason for this is the weight of the lung. Anything that is supported requires a larger pressure below it than above it to balance the downward-acting weight forces, and the lung, which is partly supported by the rib cage and diaphragm, is no exception. The result is that the pressure near the base is higher (less negative) than at the apex.

Figure 3–11 shows the way in which the volume of a portion of lung (for example, a lobe) expands as the pressure around it is decreased (compare with Fig. 3–9). The pressure inside the lung is the same as atmospheric pressure. Note that the lung is easier to inflate at low volumes than at high volumes, where it becomes stiffer. Because the expanding pressure at the base of the lung is small, this region has a small resting volume. However, because it is situated on a steep part of the pressure-volume curve, it expands well on inspiration. By contrast, the apex of the lung has a large expanding pressure, a big resting volume, and a small change in volume on inspiration.

Now when we talk of regional differences of ventilation, we mean the change in volume per unit resting volume. It is clear from Figure 3–11 that the base of the lung has both a larger change in volume and a smaller resting volume than the apex. Therefore, its ventilation is greater. Note the paradox that although the base of the lung is relatively poorly expanded compared with the apex, it is better ventilated. The same explana-

tion can be given for the large ventilation of dependent lung in both the supine and lateral positions.

A remarkable change in the distribution of ventilation occurs at low lung volumes. **FIGURE 3–12** is similar to Figure 3–11 except that it represents the situation at residual volume (that is, after a maximal expiration; *see* Fig. 3–6). Now the intrapleural pressures are less negative, because the lung is not so well expanded and the elastic recoil forces are smaller. However, the differences between the apex and base are still present because of the weight of the lung. The intrapleural pressure at the base now actually exceeds airway (atmospheric) pressure. Under these conditions, the lung at the base is not being expanded but compressed, and ventilation is impossible until the local intrapleural pressure falls below atmospheric pressure. By contrast, the apex of the lung is on a favorable part of the pressure-volume curve and ventilates well. Therefore, the normal distribution of ventilation is inverted, the upper regions ventilating better than the lower zones.

Airway Closure

The compressed region of lung at the base does not have all of its gas squeezed out. In practice, small airways, probably in the region of respiratory bronchioles (*see* Fig. 1–5), close first, thus trapping gas in the distal alveoli. This airway closure occurs only at very low lung volumes in young normal subjects. However, in elderly apparently healthy persons, airway closure in the lowermost regions of the lung occurs at higher volumes and may even be present at functional residual capacity (Fig. 3–6). The reason for this

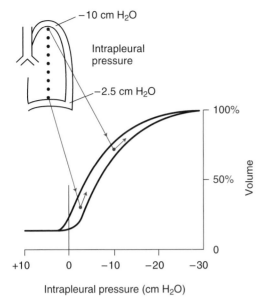

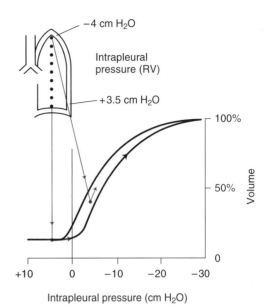

FIGURE 3–11. Explanation of the regional differences of ventilation down the lung. Because of the weight of the lung, the intrapleural pressure is less negative at the base than the apex. As a consequence, the basal lung is relatively compressed in its resting state, but expands better on inspiration than the apex.

FIGURE 3–12. Situation at residual volume. Now intrapleural pressures are less negative, and the pressure at the lung base actually exceeds airway (atmospheric) pressure. As a consequence, airway closure occurs in this region, and no gas enters with small inspirations. The alveoli at the lung base still contain some air.

is that the aging lung loses some of its elastic recoil, and intrapleural pressures therefore become less negative, thus approaching the situation shown in Figure 3–12. In these circumstances, dependent regions of the lung may be only intermittently ventilated, and this leads to defective gas exchange. A similar situation frequently develops in patients with emphysema such as Chuck in whom, again, the lung has lost some elastic recoil.

Forced Expiration

This can be measured with a simple spirometer. The *forced expiratory volume* (FEV_1) is the volume of gas exhaled in 1 second by a forced expiration from TLC. As we have seen, the *vital capacity* is the total volume of gas that can be exhaled from TLC. Because the vital capacity measured with a forced expiration is sometimes smaller than that measured with a slow expiration, the former is called the *forced vital capacity* (FVC). Table 3–1 shows that the two values in the case of Chuck were 3.1 and 3.3 liters.

FIGURE 3–13A shows a typical normal tracing. The volume exhaled in 1 second was 4.0

liters and the total volume exhaled was 5.0 liters. Therefore the ratio of FEV_1 to FVC was 80%. However, the predicted values depend on age, gender, and height (see Appendix A). The FEV can be measured over other times, such as 2 or 3 seconds, but the 1 second value is the most informative. When the subscript is omitted, the period is 1 second.

By contrast, Figure 3–13B shows the tracing obtained from Chuck, who has chronic obstructive pulmonary disease. The rate at which the air was exhaled was much slower so that only 1.3 liters were blown out in the first second. In addition, the total volume exhaled was only 3.1 liters. Therefore the FEV_1/FVC was reduced to 42%. These figures are typical of severe obstructive disease.

Figure 3–13C shows the typical pattern of a patient with severe restrictive disease, for example pulmonary fibrosis. Here the FVC was reduced to 3.1 liters, but a large percentage (90%) was exhaled in the first second. This pattern will be discussed in more detail in Chapter 5.

Another measurement which is often made on a forced expiration is the forced expiratory

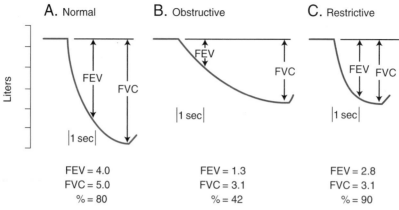

FIGURE 3–13. Forced expirations. **A.** Normal. **B.** Obstructive pattern. **C.** Restrictive pattern.

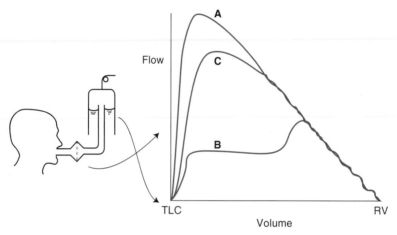

FIGURE 3–14. Flow-volume curves. **A.** A maximal inspiration was followed by a forced expiration. **B.** Expiration was initially slow and then forced. **C.** Expiratory effort was submaximal. In all three, the descending portions of the curves are almost superimposed.

flow ($FEF_{25-75\%}$). The middle half by volume of the total expiration is marked, and its duration is measured. The $FEF_{25-75\%}$ is the volume in liters divided by the time in seconds. Table 3–1 shows that the value in Chuck was $1.4 \ l \cdot sec^{-1}$. The correlation between $FEF_{25-75\%}$ and FEV_1 is generally close in patients with obstructive pulmonary disease. The changes in $FEF_{25-75\%}$ are often more striking but the range of normal values is greater.

Dynamic Compression of Airways

The changes that take place in Chuck's airways during a forced expiration are extremely important because they are a major source of his chief complaint, that is shortness of breath, and they contribute greatly to his disability. However, to understand fully what is going on requires further analysis.

Suppose a normal subject inhales to TLC and then exhales as hard as possible to residual volume (RV). We can record a *flow-volume curve* like A in **FIGURE 3–14,** which shows that flow rises very rapidly to a high value but then declines over most of the expiration. A remarkable feature of this flow-volume envelope is that it is virtually impossible to get outside it. For example, no matter whether we start exhaling slowly and then accelerate, as in B, or make a less forceful expiration as in C, the descending portion of the flow-volume curve takes virtually the same path. Therefore something powerful is limiting expiratory flow, and over most of the lung volume, flow rate is independent of effort.

We can get more information about this curious state of affairs by plotting the data in another way as shown in **FIGURE 3–15**. For this, the subject takes a *series* of maximal inspirations (or expirations) and then exhales (or inhales) fully with varying degrees of effort. If the flow rates and intrapleural pressures are plotted at the *same* lung volume for each expiration and inspiration, so-called *iso-volume pressure-flow curves* can be obtained. It can be seen that at high lung volumes, the expiratory flow rate continues to increase with effort as might be expected. However at mid or low volumes, the flow rate reaches a plateau and cannot be raised by further increases in intrapleural pressure. Therefore under these conditions, flow is *effort-independent*.

The reason for this remarkable behavior is compression of the airways by intrathoracic pressure. **FIGURE 3–16** shows schematically the forces acting across an airway within the lung.

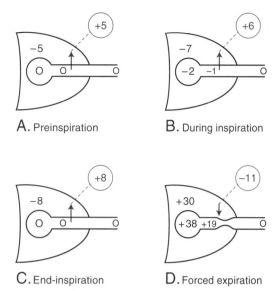

A. Preinspiration   B. During inspiration

C. End-inspiration   D. Forced expiration

FIGURE 3–16. Scheme showing why airways are compressed during a forced expiration. The pressure difference across the airway is holding it open, except during a forced expiration. (See text for details.)

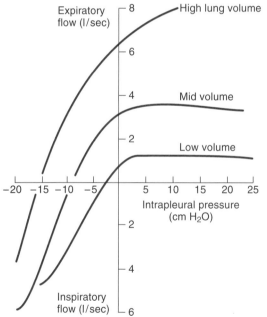

FIGURE 3–15. Isovolume pressure-flow curves drawn for three lung volumes. Each of these was obtained from a series of forced expirations and inspirations (see text). At the high lung volume, a rise in intrapleural pressure (obtained by increasing expiratory effort) results in a greater expiratory flow. However, at mid and low volumes, flow becomes independent of effort after a certain intrapleural pressure has been exceeded.

The pressure outside the airway is shown as intrapleural, although this is an oversimplification. In A, before inspiration has begun, airway pressure is everywhere zero (no flow). Since intrapleural pressure is −5 cm water, there is a pressure of 5 cm water holding the airway open. As inspiration starts (B), both intrapleural and alveolar pressure fall by 2 cm water (same lung volume as A), and flow begins. Because of the pressure drop along the airway, the pressure inside is −1 cm water, and there is now a pressure of 6 cm water holding the airway open. At end-inspiration (C), flow is again zero, and there is an airway transmural pressure of 8 cm water.

Finally, at the onset of forced expiration (D), both intrapleural pressure and alveolar pressure increase by 38 cm water (same lung volume as C). Because of the pressure drop along the airway as flow begins, there is now a pressure of 11 cm water, tending to *close* the airway. Airway compression occurs, and the downstream pressure limiting flow becomes the pressure outside the airway, or intrapleural pressure. Thus the effective driving pressure becomes alveolar minus intrapleural pressure. The basic reason is that in a collapsible tube such as the airway, the pressure inside the tube at the point of compression is the same as the pressure outside the tube, and the mouth pressure becomes immaterial (*see* Fig. 6.8, in which the same situation occurs in a blood vessel). If intrapleural pressure is raised further by increased muscular effort in an attempt to expel gas, the effective driving pressure is unaltered because the elastic recoil of the lung depends only on its volume (Fig. 3–9). Therefore flow is independent of effort.

Maximum flow decreases with lung volume (Fig. 3–14) because the difference between alveolar and intrapleural pressure decreases (Fig. 3–9), and also the airways become narrower. Also, flow is independent of the resistance of the airways downstream of the point of collapse, called the *equal pressure point*. As expiration progresses, the equal pressure point moves distally, deeper into the lung. This occurs because the resistance of the airways rises as lung volume falls, and therefore the pressure within the airways falls more rapidly with distance from the alveoli.

Several factors exaggerate this flow-limiting mechanism in Chuck. One is the loss of radial traction on the airways by lung parenchyma because of the destruction of the lung architecture (Figs. 3–2B and 3–3B). This means that the airways are more easily compressed. Another is the increased resistance of the peripheral airways which comes about because many of these have been destroyed by the emphysematous process, along with the alveolar walls. The result is that the pressure inside the airways falls more rapidly as air moves from the alveoli toward the mouth. Finally, the driving pressure (alveolar minus intrapleural) is reduced in Chuck because his lung compliance is increased. The result is that while this type of flow limitation is only seen during forced expirations in normal subjects, it may occur during the expirations of normal breathing in patients like Chuck with severe chronic obstructive pulmonary disease. This is a major factor limiting his increase in ventilation on exercise, and therefore his maximal oxygen uptake.

Arterial Blood Gases

Table 3–1 shows that Chuck's arterial P_{O_2} is only 58 mm Hg, whereas the predicted normal value is 85 mm Hg. Incidentally, you may ask why this predicted value is so much lower than Bill's in Chapter 2. The answer is that the normal value declines with age.

The reason for the reduction in arterial P_{O_2} in a patient like Chuck leads us into one of the most

difficult areas of pulmonary physiology. Clearly, the reason is not a reduction of inspired P_{O_2}, as it was in the case of Bill. Furthermore, it turns out that Chuck has adequate amounts of both ventilation and blood flow going to his lung. The basic problem is that the matching of ventilation and blood flow in different areas has been disturbed by his disease and this ventilation-perfusion inequality, as it is called, is responsible for the hypoxemia.

Ventilation-Perfusion Inequality

We can gain some insight into why the ratio of ventilation to blood flow is important in gas exchange by referring to a simple model (**FIGURE 3–17**). The model is made of glass, and is meant to represent a lung unit with an airway and a blood vessel. Powdered dye is continuously poured into the unit to represent the addition of O_2 by alveolar ventilation. Water is pumped continuously through the unit to represent the blood flow which removes the O_2. A stirrer mixes the alveolar contents, a process normally accomplished by gaseous diffusion. The key question is: what determines the concentration of dye (or O_2) in the alveolar compartment, and therefore in the effluent water (or blood)?

It is clear that both the rate at which the dye is added (ventilation) and the rate at which water is

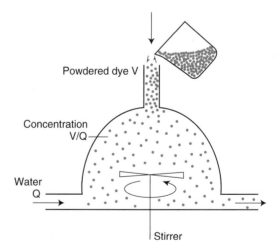

FIGURE 3–17. Model that illustrates how the ventilation-perfusion ratio determines the P_{O_2} in a lung unit. Powdered dye is added by ventilation at the rate V and removed by blood flow Q to represent the factors controlling alveolar P_{O_2}. The concentration of dye is given by V/Q.

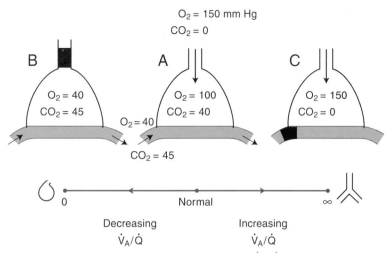

FIGURE 3–18. Effect of altering the ventilation-perfusion ratio ($\dot{V}A/\dot{Q}$) on the P_{O_2} and P_{CO_2} in a lung unit.

pumped (blood flow) will affect the concentration of dye in the model. What may not be intuitively clear is that the concentration of dye is determined by the ratio of these rates. In other words, if dye is added at the rate of V g · min⁻¹ and water is pumped through at Q l · min⁻¹, then the concentration of dye in the alveolar compartment and effluent water is V/Q g · l⁻¹.

In exactly the same way, the concentration of oxygen (or better, the P_{O_2}) in any lung unit is determined by the ratio of ventilation to blood flow; and this applies not only to O_2 but CO_2, N_2, and any other gas that is present under steady-state conditions. This is the reason why the ventilation-perfusion ratio plays such a key role in pulmonary gas exchange.

Now let's take a closer look at the way alterations in the ventilation-perfusion ratio of a lung unit affect its gas exchange. **FIGURE 3–18A** shows the P_{O_2} and P_{CO_2} in a unit with a normal ventilation-perfusion ratio of about 1 (compare with Fig. 1–6). The inspired air has a P_{O_2} of 150 mm Hg (*see* Fig. 2–2) and a P_{CO_2} of zero. The mixed venous blood entering the unit normally has a P_{O_2} of 40 mm Hg and P_{CO_2} of 45 mm Hg. The alveolar P_{O_2} of 100 mm Hg is determined by a balance between the addition of O_2 by ventilation and its removal by blood flow (*see* Fig. 2–2). The normal alveolar P_{O_2} of 40 mm Hg is set similarly.

Now suppose that the ventilation-perfusion ratio of the unit is gradually reduced by obstructing its ventilation, leaving its blood flow unchanged (Fig. 3–18B). It is clear that the O_2 in the unit will fall and the CO_2 will rise, although

the relative changes of these two are not immediately obvious. However, we can easily predict what will eventually happen when the ventilation is completely abolished (ventilation-perfusion ratio of zero). Now the O_2 and CO_2 of alveolar gas and end-capillary blood must be the same as those of mixed venous blood. (In practice, completely obstructed units eventually collapse, but we can neglect such long-term effects at the moment.) We are assuming that what happens in one unit out of a very large number does not affect the composition of mixed venous blood.

Suppose, however, that the ventilation-perfusion ratio is increased by gradually obstructing blood flow (Fig. 3–18C). Now the O_2 rises and the CO_2 falls, eventually reaching the composition of inspired gas when blood flow is abolished (ventilation-perfusion ratio of infinity). Thus as the ventilation-perfusion ratio of the unit is altered, its gas composition approaches that of either mixed venous blood or inspired gas.

Now, in Chuck's lung the destruction of the normal architecture (Figs. 3–2B and 3–3B) means that there are areas of very different ventilation-perfusion ratios scattered more or less randomly throughout the lung, and as a consequence, it is difficult to understand the effects on gas exchange. However, it turns out that in the normal upright lung, the differences of ventilation-perfusion ratio are much less extreme, but they are distributed in an orderly way. In fact, we can learn a good deal about the effects of ventilation-perfusion inequality on gas

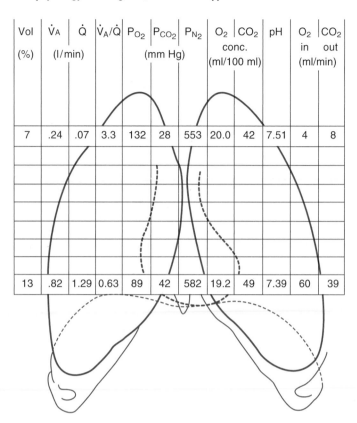

Vol (%)	$\dot{V}_A$ (l/min)	$\dot{Q}$ (l/min)	$\dot{V}_A/\dot{Q}$	P_{O_2} (mm Hg)	P_{CO_2} (mm Hg)	P_{N_2} (mm Hg)	O_2 conc. (ml/100 ml)	CO_2 conc. (ml/100 ml)	pH	O_2 in (ml/min)	CO_2 out (ml/min)
7	.24	.07	3.3	132	28	553	20.0	42	7.51	4	8
13	.82	1.29	0.63	89	42	582	19.2	49	7.39	60	39

FIGURE 3–19. Regional differences in gas exchange down the normal lung. The lung is divided into a series of imaginary horizontal slices but only the uppermost and lowermost values are shown for clarity. (See text for details.)

exchange by looking at the pattern in the normal lung. This is shown in **FIGURE 3–19**. Here the lung is divided into a series of imaginary horizontal slices but only the values in the uppermost and lowermost slices in the lung are shown. Between these extremes there is a gradual change but the values are not shown on the diagram because it would become too crowded.

The left-most column shows that the volume of a slice of lung is somewhat less near the apex than the base, simply because of the shape of the lung. The next column shows that ventilation is less at the top of the lung than at the bottom, as we saw earlier in this chapter (Fig. 3–10). The next column shows that blood flow is very uneven, with the apex of the lung only barely perfused. Again, the culprit is gravity, and the mechanism will be discussed in Chapter 6. The net result of these differences of ventilation and blood flow is that the ventilation-perfusion ratio is high near the top of the lung and relatively low near the bottom.

Now we have already seen that the ventilation-perfusion ratio determines regional gas exchange. As Figure 3–18 implies, the high ventilation-perfusion ratio at the top of the lung means that the P_{O_2} there will be relatively high (compared with the bottom), and the P_{CO_2} will be relatively low. The difference in P_{N_2} in the next column comes about because the sum of the partial pressures must add up to atmospheric pressure. The O_2 and CO_2 dissociation curves (*see* Figs. 1–14 and 1–17) mean that the O_2 and CO_2 concentrations in the blood draining from the lung units at the top and bottom of the lung are different. The fact that the P_{CO_2} is relatively low at the top of the lung means that the pH there is relatively high (*see* Fig. 2–4). The differences in O_2 uptake and CO_2 output shown in the last two columns are caused by both the differences of P_{O_2} and P_{CO_2}, and the differences of blood flow and ventilation.

These regional differences of gas exchange have some clinical consequences. For example, the tendency for adult tuberculosis to occur in the apex of the lung can be explained by the high P_{O_2} there. The reason is that tubercle bacillus thrives better in a P_{O_2} of 130 than one of 90. However, while these regional differences of gas exchange are of interest, more important to the body as a whole is whether mismatching of ventilation and blood flow affects the overall gas exchange of the lung, that is, its ability to take up O_2 and put out CO_2. It turns out that a lung with ventilation-perfusion inequality is not able to transfer as much O_2 and CO_2 as a lung that is uniformly ventilated and perfused, other things being equal. In addition, if the same amounts of gas are being transferred (because these are set by the metabolic demands of the body), a lung with ventilation-perfusion inequality cannot maintain as high an arterial P_{O_2} or as low an arterial P_{CO_2} as a homogeneous lung, again with other things being equal.

The reason why a lung with uneven ventilation and blood flow has difficulty oxygenating arterial blood can be illustrated by looking at the differences down the upright lung **(FIGURE 3–20)**. The P_{O_2} at the apex is some 40 mm higher than at the base of the lung (compare Fig. 3–19). However, the major share of the blood leaving the lung comes from the lower zones, where the P_{O_2} is low. This has the result of depressing the arterial P_{O_2}. By contrast, the expired alveolar ventilation comes more uniformly from apex and base, because the differences of ventilation are much less than those for blood flow (Fig. 3–19). By the same reasoning, the arterial P_{CO_2} will be elevated since it is higher at the base of the lung than at the apex (Fig. 3–19).

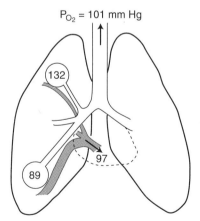

P_{O_2} = 101 mm Hg

132

97

89

FIGURE 3–20. Depression of the arterial P_{O_2} by ventilation-perfusion inequality. In this diagram of the upright lung, only two groups of alveoli at the top and bottom are shown. The relative sizes of the airways and blood vessels indicate their relative ventilations and blood flows. Because most of the blood comes from the oxygenated base, depression of the blood P_{O_2} is inevitable.

An additional reason why uneven ventilation and blood flow depress the arterial P_{O_2} is shown in **FIGURE 3–21**. This depicts three groups of alveoli with low, normal, and high ventilation-perfusion ratios. The O_2 concentrations of the effluent blood are 16.0, 19.5, and 20.0 ml $\cdot$ dl^{-1}, respectively. As a result, the units with the high ventilation-perfusion ratio add relatively little oxygen to the blood compared with the decrement caused by the alveoli with the low ventilation-perfusion ratio. Therefore, the mixed capillary blood has a lower O_2 concentration than that from units with a normal ventilation-perfusion ratio. This can be explained by the very nonlinear shape of the O_2 dissociation curve (*see* Fig. 1–14), which means that, although units with a high ventilation-perfusion ratio have a relatively high P_{O_2}, this does not increase the O_2 concentration of their blood very much. This additional reason for the depression of P_{O_2} in the blood does not apply to the elevation of the P_{CO_2}, because the CO_2 dissociation curve is almost linear in the working range (*see* Fig. 1–17).

The net result of these mechanisms is a depression of the arterial P_{O_2} below that of the mixed alveolar P_{O_2}. In the upright normal lung this difference is of trivial magnitude, being only about 4 mm Hg as a result of ventilation-perfusion inequality (Fig. 3–20). Its development is described here only to illustrate how uneven ventilation and blood flow *must* result in depression of the arterial P_{O_2}. In lung disease, the lowering of arterial P_{O_2} by this mechanism can be much greater, as we shall shortly see in Chuck's case.

Distributions of Ventilation-Perfusion Ratios

It is possible to obtain information about the distribution of ventilation-perfusion ratios in patients, such as Chuck, who have lung disease by infusing into a peripheral vein a mixture of inert gases having a range of solubilities, and measuring the concentrations of the gases in arterial blood and expired gas. The details of this technique are too complex to be described here, and it is mainly used for research purposes rather than in the pulmonary function laboratory. The technique returns a distribution of ventilation and blood flow plotted against ventilation-perfusion ratio with 50 compartments equally spaced on a log scale.

FIGURE 3–21. Additional reason for the depression of arterial P_{O_2} by mismatching of ventilation and blood flow. The lung units with a high ventilation-perfusion ratio add relatively little oxygen to the blood, compared with the decrement caused by alveoli with a low ventilation-perfusion ratio.

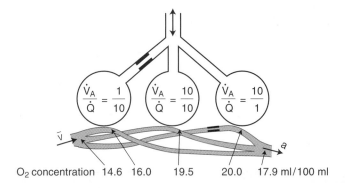

O_2 concentration 14.6 16.0   19.5   20.0   17.9 ml/100 ml

FIGURE 3–22 shows a typical result from a young healthy subject such as Ann or Bill. All the ventilation and blood flow go to compartments close to the normal ventilation-perfusion ratio of about 1.0 (compare with Fig. 1–6), and in particular, there is no blood flow to any unventilated compartment (shunt). However, **FIGURE 3–23** shows that the distribution for Chuck is very different. Although much of the ventilation and blood flow go to compartments where the ventilation-perfusion ratio is near normal, considerable blood flow is going to compartments with ventilation-perfusion ratios of between 0.03 and 0.3. Blood from these units will be oxygen-ated poorly and will depress the arterial P_{O_2}. These lung units are presumably those supplied by partly obstructed airways caused by retained secretions or swelling of the airway walls; these are typical features of chronic bronchitis. There is also excessive ventilation to lung units with ventilation-perfusion ratios up to 10. These units are inefficient at eliminating CO_2. These overventilated but underperfused units may be in regions of the lung shown, for example, in Figures 3–2B and 3–3B where alveolar walls have been destroyed and many of the capillaries have been obliterated but ventilation still occurs.

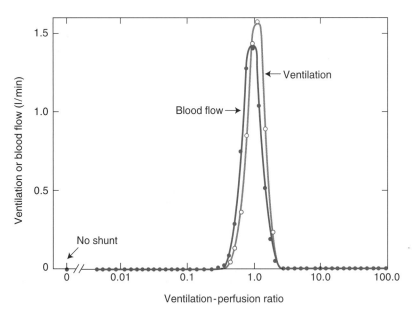

FIGURE 3–22. Distribution of ventilation-perfusion ratios in a young, normal subject. Note the narrow dispersion of both ventilation and blood flow and the absence of blood flow to unventilated areas (shunt).

Measurement of Ventilation-Perfusion Inequality

How can we assess the amount of ventilation-perfusion inequality in a diseased lung? The inert gas technique described in the last section is available in specialized centers, but in most instances we turn to indices based on the resulting impairment of gas exchange.

A useful measurement is the *alveolar-arterial P_{O_2} difference*. This is obtained by subtracting the arterial P_{O_2} from the so-called "ideal" alveolar P_{O_2}. The latter is the P_{O_2} that the lung *would* have if there were no ventilation-perfusion inequality and the lung was exchanging gas at the same respiratory exchange ratio as the real lung. It is derived from the alveolar gas equation:

$$P_{A_{O_2}} = P_{I_{O_2}} - \frac{P_{A_{CO_2}}}{R} + F$$

The arterial P_{CO_2} is used for the alveolar value. As in our discussion of Bill, we can neglect the small correction factor F.

Let's apply this equation to Chuck's blood gases. The inspired P_{O_2} while breathing air at sea level is 149 mm Hg (*see* Fig. 2–2). His arterial P_{CO_2} from Table 3–1 is 49 and, assuming an R

value of 0.8, this means that the alveolar P_{O_2} is given by:

$$149 - \frac{49}{0.8}$$
$$= 88 \text{ mm Hg}$$

Since his arterial P_{O_2} from Table 3–1 is 58 mm Hg, the alveolar-arterial P_{O_2} difference is 30 mm Hg. This is a very high and abnormal value confirming the existence of ventilation-perfusion inequality.

Arterial P_{CO_2}

Table 3–1 shows that Chuck's arterial P_{CO_2} is 49 mm Hg. The normal value is 40 mm Hg, so his value is abnormally high. The reason for the increase is ventilation-perfusion inequality, just as this is the reason for the reduced arterial P_{O_2}. However, the mechanism in the case of CO_2 frequently causes confusion and warrants additional discussion.

Imagine a lung that is uniformly ventilated and perfused and that is transferring normal amounts of O_2 and CO_2. Suppose that in some magical way, the matching of ventilation and blood flow is suddenly disturbed while everything else remains unchanged. What happens to

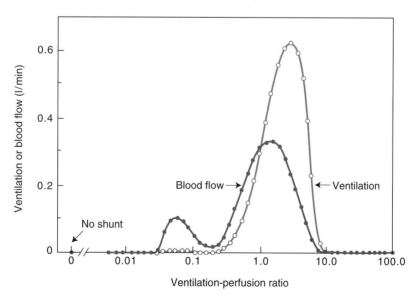

FIGURE 3–23. Distribution of ventilation-perfusion ratios in Chuck, who has chronic bronchitis and emphysema. There is increased blood flow to lung units with very low ventilation-perfusion ratios. There is also increased ventilation to units with abnormally high ventilation-perfusion ratios.

gas exchange? It transpires that the effect of this "pure" ventilation-perfusion inequality (that is, everything else held constant) is to reduce *both* the O_2 uptake and CO_2 output of the lung. In other words, the lung becomes less efficient as a gas exchanger for both gases. Therefore, mismatching ventilation and blood flow must cause both a reduced P_{O_2} and an increased P_{CO_2} (CO_2 retention, or hypercapnia), other things being equal.

Confusion arises because patients like Chuck with undoubted ventilation-perfusion inequality often have a normal arterial P_{CO_2}. The reason for this is that whenever the chemoreceptors (*see* Figs. 2–6 and 2–7) sense a rising P_{CO_2} there is an increase in the output of the respiratory centers which increases the action of the respiratory muscles. The consequent increase in ventilation to the alveoli often returns the arterial P_{CO_2} to normal. However, these patients can only maintain a normal P_{CO_2} at the expense of this increased ventilation to their alveoli; the ventilation in excess of what they would normally require is sometimes referred to as *wasted ventilation* and is necessary because the lung units with abnormally high ventilation-perfusion ratios are inefficient at eliminating CO_2. Such units are said to constitute an *alveolar dead space*.

While the increase in ventilation to a lung with ventilation-perfusion inequality is usually effective at reducing the arterial P_{CO_2}, it is much less effective at increasing the arterial P_{O_2}. The reason for the different behavior of the two gases lies in the shapes of the CO_2 and O_2 dissociation curves. As Figure 1–17 (*see* Chapter 1) shows, the CO_2 dissociation curve is almost straight in the working range, with the result that an increase in ventilation will raise the CO_2 output of lung units with both high and low ventilation-perfusion ratios. By contrast, the almost flat top of the O_2 dissociation curve (*see* Fig. 1–14) means that only units with moderately low ventilation-perfusion ratios will benefit appreciably from the increased ventilation. Those units that are very high on the oxygen dissociation curve (high ventilation-perfusion ratio) increase the O_2 concentration of their effluent blood very little (Fig. 3–21). Those units that have a very low ventilation-perfusion ratio continue to put out blood with an O_2 concentration close to that of mixed venous blood. The net result is that the mixed arterial P_{O_2} rises only modestly, and some hypoxemia always remains.

Sometimes the increased arterial P_{CO_2} in patients like Chuck is attributed to "hypoventilation." However, this is misleading. As described above, the primary cause is ventilation-perfusion inequality, and indeed patients like Chuck are moving *more* air into their alveoli (and into their lung generally) than normal subjects. Hypoventilation *can* cause an increased arterial P_{CO_2} just as hyperventilation reduced the arterial P_{CO_2} in Bill at high altitude (*see* Fig. 2–2). Diseases in which hypoventilation increases the arterial P_{CO_2} are discussed in Chapter 9. However, it is misleading to attribute the CO_2 retention in a patient like Chuck to hypoventilation.

Arterial pH

As Table 3–1 shows, Chuck's arterial pH was 7.36, that is there was a mild acidosis. Since this was caused by an increased arterial P_{CO_2}, the mechanism is respiratory acidosis. By referring to the Davenport diagram shown in Figure 2–4 (*see* Chapter 2), we can see that the pH was not reduced as much as we would expect from a P_{CO_2} of 49 mm Hg if this were a pure respiratory acidosis with the point moving to the left along the normal blood buffer line. Therefore there must have been some renal compensation with conservation of bicarbonate with the result that the pH was returned some way toward the normal value of 7.4. This means that his acid-base status is best described as partially compensated respiratory acidosis.

Exercise Test

This showed that Chuck's maximal oxygen consumption was only 1.2 $1 \cdot min^{-1}$, a grossly reduced value. Recall that Ann's $\dot{V}_{O_2}max$ was 3.5 $1 \cdot min^{-1}$. There are several reasons for the reduced exercise capacity. One of the most important was the dynamic compression of the airways during expiration (Fig. 3–16). The result is that the extent to which he could increase his ventilation during exercise was severely limited. In addition, however, his lung was very inefficient as a gas exchanger, as we can see from the reduced arterial P_{O_2}, the increased arterial P_{CO_2}, and the increased alveolar-arterial P_{O_2} difference. Another factor was the pulmonary hypertension and resultant right heart failure which limited the increase in cardiac output during exercise, and therefore the delivery of oxygen to the exercising muscles.

☐ TREATMENT AND PROGRESS

Oxygen was given to improve the hypoxemia, and bronchodilators reduced his airway obstruction to some extent; bronchodilators will be discussed in Chapter 4. Diuretics were administered to reduce the amount of peripheral edema.

As we saw earlier, Chuck was readmitted to the hospital 6 months later with an acute chest infection, a common occurrence in patients with chronic bronchitis. The rales (crackles) in his chest developed as a result of retained secretions. Worsening ventilation-perfusion inequality reduced his arterial P_{O_2} to 42 mm Hg, increased his arterial P_{CO_2} to 55 mm Hg, and resulted in a more severe respiratory acidosis with a pH of 7.30. Unfortunately, his condition deteriorated despite therapy, his arterial P_{CO_2} rose to 65 mm Hg, and he subsequently died. The increase in arterial P_{CO_2} is often referred to as respiratory failure (*see* Chapter 9).

☐ PATHOGENESIS

The mechanisms responsible for chronic obstructive pulmonary disease are still not fully understood, and this is an active area of research. However, there is no doubt that a major factor in the development of Chuck's disease was the long history of cigarette smoking. This caused chronic bronchitis through repeated exposure of the airways to noxious cigarette smoke. It is also very likely that Chuck's emphysema was caused in large part by cigarette smoking. A clue to the pathogenesis of this condition is that patients with a congenital deficiency of α_1-antitrypsin often develop emphysema at a relatively early age, even when there is no smoking history. This suggests that the disease is related in some way to protease activity in the lung.

A current hypothesis is that excessive amounts of the enzyme, lysosomal elastase, are released from neutrophils in the lung. This results in the destruction of elastin, an important structural protein of the lung. In addition, neutrophil elastase cleaves type IV collagen, and there is evidence that this molecule is important in determining the strength of the thin blood-gas barrier (*see* Fig. 1–7) which makes up a major part of the pulmonary capillary wall. This may lead to destruction of the alveolar wall. Experimental animals that have neutrophil elastase instilled into their airways develop histological changes that are similar in many respects to emphysema.

The exact role of cigarette smoking is still unclear but it may work by stimulating macrophages to produce neutrophil chemoattractants such as C5a, or by reducing the activity of elastase inhibitors. In addition, many neutrophils are normally marginated (trapped) in the lung, and this process is exaggerated by cigarette smoking, which also activates trapped leukocytes. This is a very active area of current research.

Finally, because of the clear evidence that cigarette smoking is a major etiological factor in chronic obstructive pulmonary disease, as well as a number of other lung and heart diseases, physicians and medical students have a clear responsibility to try to reduce the amount of their patients' cigarette smoking.

Questions

For each question, choose the one best answer. (For answers, see p. 150.)

1. Features of emphysema (in the absence of chronic bronchitis) include all of the following EXCEPT:
   A. Loss of alveolar walls
   B. Hypertrophy of bronchial mucous glands
   C. Loss of radial traction around extra-alveolar blood vessels
   D. Reduced lung elastic recoil
   E. Loss of pulmonary capillaries

2. Which of the following cannot be measured with a simple spirometer and stopwatch?
   A. Vital capacity
   B. Tidal volume
   C. Total ventilation
   D. Residual volume
   E. Breathing frequency

3. Which of the following is typically decreased in a patient with emphysema?
   A. Total lung capacity
   B. Residual volume
   C. Functional residual capacity
   D. Vital capacity
   E. Lung compliance

4. A normal subject is connected to a 1.5-liter volume rubber bag containing 9% helium and rapidly rebreathes over 10 seconds until the helium concentration in the bag and lung are the same. If the final helium concentration is 3% and the subject is at functional residual capacity when he is connected to the bag, the FRC (in liters) is:
   A. 2
   B. 2.5
   C. 3
   D. 3.5
   E. 4

5. The following statements about the pressure-volume behavior of lung are true EXCEPT:
   A. The pressure-volume curve is different during inflation compared with deflation.
   B. Compliance is the volume change per unit pressure change.
   C. The compliance of the normal human lung is about $0.2 \, l \cdot cm \, H_2O^{-1}$.
   D. If intrapleural pressure is raised above alveolar pressure, the alveoli become airless.
   E. In a patient, esophageal pressure can be used as a measure of intrapleural pressure.

6. A patient with emphysema is found to have an abnormally low airflow rate during the middle half of a forced expiration. All of the following factors contribute to the low rate EXCEPT:
   A. Reduced strength of diaphragmatic contraction
   B. Reduced pressure difference between alveolar and intrapleural spaces
   C. Reduced radial traction on intrapulmonary airways
   D. Increased resistance of small airways because some have been destroyed
   E. Increased lung compliance

7. Suppose the ventilation-perfusion ratio of a lung unit is gradually decreased by partial obstruction of its airway. In the lung unit all of the following occur EXCEPT:
   A. Alveolar P_{O_2} falls.
   B. P_{CO_2} of end-capillary blood rises.
   C. pH of end-capillary blood falls.
   D. Base excess of end-capillary blood falls.
   E. O_2 saturation of end-capillary blood falls.

8. A patient breathing air has an arterial P_{O_2} of 49 mm Hg, P_{CO_2} of 48 mm Hg, and respiratory exchange ratio of 0.8. The approximate alveolar-arterial difference for P_{O_2} in mm Hg is:
   A. 20
   B. 25
   C. 30

D. 35
E. 40

9. **The laboratory reports the arterial blood gases in a patient with severe lung disease as: Po_2 60 mm Hg, Pco_2 110 mm Hg, and pH 7.20. All of the following are true EXCEPT:**
   A. There is hypoxemia.
   B. There is CO_2 retention.
   C. There is respiratory acidosis.
   D. There is some renal compensation for the acidosis.
   E. The patient is breathing air.

10. **All of the following statements are true about the pathogenesis of emphysema EXCEPT:**
   A. Neutrophil elastase attacks elastin fibers in the alveolar wall.
   B. Neutrophil elastase can cleave type IV collagen.
   C. Cigarette smoking is responsible for more disease than atmospheric pollution.
   D. Patients with α_1-antitrypsin deficiency who do not smoke cigarettes commonly develop emphysema.
   E. The earliest pathological changes occur in the small bronchi.

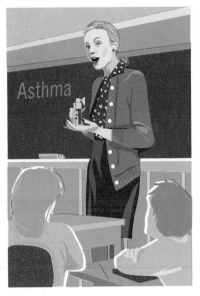

Chapter 4

Asthma

☐ Debra is a 30-year-old school teacher who has had asthma for the past 20 years. This is characterized by periods of severe shortness of breath, particularly in the spring when the pollen count is high, but also during exercise or exposure to cold air. First we look at the pathological changes in the airways. We then discuss patterns of airflow in the lung, the pressures during the breathing cycle, the factors determining airway resistance, uneven ventilation, the pathogenesis of asthma, and the principles of action of bronchoactive drugs.

☐ CLINICAL FINDINGS

Debra is a 30-year-old school teacher whose main complaint is shortness of breath which changes considerably in severity from time to time. She is particularly affected in the spring when the pollen count is high. She first began to notice problems with breathing at the age of 9 when a diagnosis of asthma was made. Since then, she has had frequent attacks of wheezing, accompanied by runny nose and watery eyes, especially in the spring. She likes to play tennis, but often exercise brings on an attack. Another provocative factor is cold air when she goes outside in the winter. She also tends to have attacks when she is under stress, for example at examination times. Three years ago, Debra experienced a severe attack which responded poorly to bronchodilator drugs and inhaled steroids. She became exhausted, dehydrated, and very anxious. She eventually recovered but was hospitalized for 3 days. Apart from her asthma, Debra's health is good. She has never smoked cigarettes. Her mother also had asthma.

On examination during a typical attack, Debra was dyspneic, orthopneic, and anxious. The accessory muscles of respiration were active. The lungs were hyperinflated, and musical rhonchi could be heard in all areas by ausculta-

tion. The pulse was rapid, and pulsus paradoxus was present (marked fall in systolic and pulse pressure during inspiration). The sputum was scant and viscid. The chest radiograph revealed hyperinflation but was otherwise normal. No abnormalities were found in other systems.

☐ PATHOLOGY

It was not possible to see the structure of Debra's lung but the pathology of asthma has been studied extensively. The airways have hypertrophied smooth muscle that contracts during an attack, causing bronchoconstriction (FIGURE 4–1B). In addition, there is hypertrophy of bronchial mucous glands, inflammation and edema of the bronchial wall, and extensive cellular infiltrations especially by eosinophils. The mucus is abnormal; it is thick, tenacious, and slow-moving. In severe cases, many of the airways are occluded by mucous plugs, some of which may be coughed up in the sputum. The sputum is typically scant and white. Subepithelial fibrosis is commonly seen in chronic asthma. In uncomplicated asthma, there is no destruction of alveolar walls, as in emphysema, and there are no copious purulent bronchial secretions, as in chronic bronchitis.

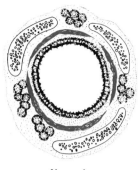

Normal

A

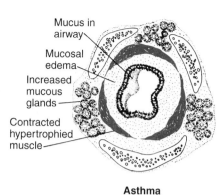

Mucus in
airway

Mucosal
edema

Increased
mucous
glands

Contracted
hypertrophied
muscle

Asthma

B

FIGURE 4–1. Bronchial wall in asthma (diagrammatic). Note the hypertrophied, contracted smooth muscle, edema, mucous gland hypertrophy, and secretion in the lumen.

☐ PULMONARY FUNCTION TESTS

As was the case with Chuck in Chapter 3, the changes in pulmonary function generally follow clearly from the pathology.

Ventilatory Capacity and Mechanics

During an attack, all indices of expiratory flow rate are reduced significantly, including the FEV_1, FEV/FVC% (*see* Fig. 3–13), and $FEF_{25-75\%}$. The FVC is also usually reduced because airways close prematurely toward the end of a maximal expiration. Between attacks, some impairment of ventilatory capacity can usually be demonstrated, although the patient may claim to feel normal. The pattern of a forced expiration is often very similar to that seen in chronic obstructive pulmonary disease (*see* Fig. 3–13B).

The response of these indices of expiratory flow rate to bronchodilator drugs is of great importance in asthma **(FIGURE 4–2)**. They can be tested by administering 0.5% albuterol by aerosol from a nebulizer for 2 minutes. Typically, all indices increase substantially when a bronchodilator is administered to a patient during an attack, and the change is a valuable measure of the responsiveness of the airways. The extent of the increase varies according to the severity of the disease. In *status asthmaticus* as Debra had when she was hospitalized for 3 days, little change in the flow rates may be seen because the bronchi have become unresponsive. Again, patients in remission may show only

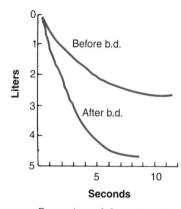

FIGURE 4–2. Examples of forced expirations before and after bronchodilator *(b.d.)* therapy in a patient with bronchial asthma.

minor improvement, although generally there is some.

In addition to plotting volume against time during a forced expiration (*see* Fig. 3–13), flow-volume curves are often measured in patients with obstructive and restrictive lung disease. Examples are shown in **FIGURE 4–3**. After administration of a bronchodilator, flows are higher at all lung volumes, and the whole curve may shift as the TLC and RV are reduced. Note that although Figure 4–3 shows changes in TLC and RV, this information is not available from a simple flow-volume curve.

Static lung volumes are increased and remarkably high values for FRC and TLC during asthma attacks have been reported. The increased RV is caused by premature airway closure toward the end of a maximal expiration as a result of the increased smooth muscle tone, edema and inflammation of the airway walls, and abnormal secretions. The cause of the increased FRC and TLC is not fully understood. However, there is some loss of elastic recoil in these patients, and the pressure-volume curve is shifted upward and to the left (**FIGURE 4–4**). The pressure-volume curve tends to return toward normal after administration of a bronchodilator. It is possible that changes in the surface tension of the alveolar lining layer are partly responsible for the altered elastic properties (*see* Chapter 6). The increase in lung volume tends to decrease the resistance of the airways by increasing the radial traction exerted by the surrounding lung parenchyma. The FRC measured by the body plethysmograph is usually considerably larger than that found by helium dilution, reflecting the presence of occluded airways or the delayed equilibration of poorly ventilated areas.

Gas Exchange

Arterial hypoxemia is common in asthma and is caused by ventilation-perfusion inequality as was

discussed in Chapter 3. In view of the pathological changes in the airways (Fig. 4–1), it is not surprising that there is much uneven ventilation. However, there is also uneven blood flow, some of which may be caused by hypoxic pulmonary vasoconstriction in regions of the lung where the ventilation has been reduced by the airway changes. Hypoxic pulmonary vasoconstriction is dealt with in Chapter 6. It is also possible that mediators released during the asthmatic process (see below) constrict some of the blood vessels as well as the airways. The alveolar-arterial P_{O_2} difference is typically increased as in chronic obstructive pulmonary disease.

An example of a distribution of ventilation-perfusion ratios in a young person with asthma is shown in **FIGURE 4–5** (compare with Fig. 3–23). This patient had only mild symptoms at the time of the measurement. However, the distribution was strikingly different from the normal distribution shown in Figure 3–22. Note especially the bimodal distribution with a considerable amount of the total blood flow (approximately 25%) going to units with low ventilation-perfusion ratios (approximately 0.1). This ac-

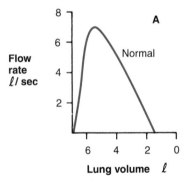

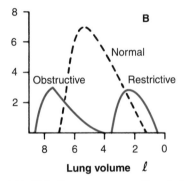

FIGURE 4–3. Expiratory flow-volume curves. **A.** Normal. **B.** This figure contrasts the obstructive and restrictive patterns (compare with Fig. 3-14).

FIGURE 4–4. Pressure-volume curves of the lung. The curves for emphysema and asthma (during bronchospasm) are shifted upward and to the left (increased compliance), whereas those for rheumatic valve disease and interstitial fibrosis are flattened (reduced compliance).

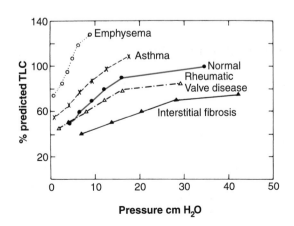

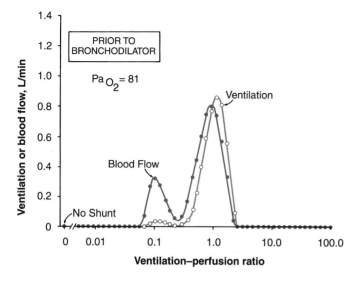

FIGURE 4–5. Distribution of ventilation-perfusion ratios in a patient with asthma. Note the bimodal appearance with approximately 24% of the total blood flow going to units with ventilation-perfusion ratios in the region of 0.1 (compare with Fig. 3-23).

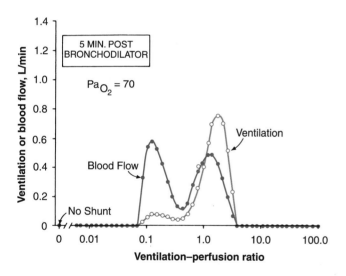

FIGURE 4–6. Measurements from the same patient as in Figure 4-5 after the administration of the bronchodilator, isoproterenol, by aerosol. Note the increase in blood flow to the units with low ventilation-perfusion ratios and the corresponding fall in arterial P_{O_2}.

counts for the patient's mild hypoxemia, the arterial P_{O_2} being 81 mm Hg. However, there was no pure shunt (blood flow to unventilated alveoli), a surprising finding in view of the mucous plugging of airways which is a feature of the disease.

When this patient was given the bronchodilator, isoproterenol, by aerosol there was a substantial increase in forced expiratory flow. Thus, there was some relief of the bronchospasm. The changes in the distribution of ventilation-perfusion ratios are shown in **FIGURE 4–6**. The blood flow to the low $\dot{V}_A/\dot{Q}$ alveoli increased from approximately 25 to 50% of the total flow, resulting in a fall in arterial P_{O_2} from 81 to 70 mm Hg. The mean $\dot{V}_A/\dot{Q}$ of the low mode

increased slightly from 0.10 to 0.14, indicating that the ventilation to these units increased slightly more than their blood flow.

Many bronchodilators decrease the arterial P_{O_2} in persons with asthma. The mechanism of the increased hypoxemia is apparently relief of vasoconstriction in poorly ventilated areas. This vasoconstriction presumably results from the release of mediators like the bronchoconstriction. However, in practice, the favorable effects of the drugs on airway resistance far exceed the disadvantages of the mild additional hypoxemia.

The absence of shunt, that is blood flow to unventilated lung units, in Figures 4–5 and 4–6 is striking because persons with asthma examined at autopsy have mucous plugs in many of their airways. Presumably, the explanation is collateral ventilation that reaches lung situated behind completely closed bronchioles. This is discussed later (*see* Fig. 4–13C). The same mechanism probably occurs in many patients with chronic bronchitis because they also typically do not have a shunt (*see* Fig. 3–23) but probably some airways are completely occluded by retained secretions.

The arterial P_{CO_2} in patients with asthma is typically normal or low, at least until late in the disease. The P_{CO_2} is prevented from rising by increased ventilation to the alveoli in the face of the ventilation-perfusion inequality (see the discussion of arterial P_{CO_2} in the patient with chronic obstructive pulmonary disease in Chapter 3). In many patients with asthma, the P_{CO_2} may be in the middle or low 30s, possibly as a result of stimulation of the peripheral chemoreceptors by the hypoxemia, or stimulation of intrapulmonary receptors. In status asthmaticus, the arterial P_{CO_2} may begin to rise and the pH to fall. This is an ominous development that denotes impending respiratory failure and signals the need for urgent and intensive treatment.

☐ PHYSIOLOGY AND PATHOPHYSIOLOGY OF THE AIRWAYS

The major functional abnormalities in Debra's lung are in the airways. To understand fully what is going on we need to discuss the principles of airflow through the airways. The anatomy of the airways was briefly reviewed in Chapter 1 (*see* Figs. 1–4 and 1–5).

Airflow Through Tubes

If air flows through a tube **(FIGURE 4–7)**, a difference of pressure exists between the ends. The pressure difference depends on the rate and pattern of flow. At low flow rates, stream lines are parallel to the sides of the tube (Fig. 4–7A). This is known as *laminar flow*. As flow rate is increased, unsteadiness develops, especially at branches. Here, separation of the stream lines from the wall may occur with the formation of local eddies (Fig. 4–7B). This is sometimes referred to as *transitional flow*. At still higher flow rates, complete disorganization of the stream lines is seen; this is *turbulence* (Fig. 4–7C).

The pressure-flow characteristics for *laminar flow* were first described by the French physician Poiseuille. In straight circular tubes, the volume flow rate ($\dot{V}$) is given by:

$$\dot{V} = \frac{P\pi r^4}{8nl}$$

where P is the driving pressure (ΔP in Fig. 4–7A); r, radius; n, viscosity; and l, length. It can be seen that the flow rate is proportional to the driving pressure, or $P = K\dot{V}$. Since flow resistance (R) is driving pressure divided by flow, rearrangement of the equation above gives:

$$R = \frac{8nl}{\pi r^4}$$

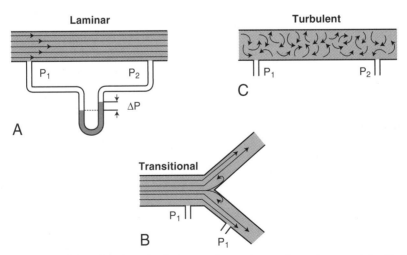

FIGURE 4–7. Patterns of airflow in tubes. In **A**, the flow is laminar; in **B**, it is transitional with eddy formation at branches; and in **C**, it is turbulent. Resistance is ($P_1 - P_2$)/flow.

Note the critical importance of the tube radius: if the radius is halved, the resistance increases 16-fold! However, doubling the length only doubles the resistance, other things being equal. Note also that the viscosity of the gas, but not its density, affects the pressure-flow relationship in pure laminar flow.

Another feature of laminar flow when this is fully developed is that the gas in the center of the tube moves twice as fast as the average velocity. Therefore, a spike of rapidly moving gas travels down the axis of the tube (Fig. 4–7A). This changing velocity across the diameter of the tube is known as the *velocity profile*.

Turbulent flow has different properties. Here the pressure is not proportional to the flow rate but, approximately, to its square: $P = K \dot{V}^2$. In addition, the viscosity of the gas becomes relatively unimportant, but an increase in gas density increases the pressure drop for a given flow. Turbulent flow does not have the very high axial flow velocity that is characteristic of laminar flow.

Whether flow will be laminar or turbulent depends to a large extent on the Reynolds number (Re). This is given by:

$$Re = \frac{2rvd}{n}$$

where d is density; v, average velocity; r, radius; and n, viscosity. Because density and velocity are in the numerator, and viscosity is in the denominator, the expression gives the ratio of inertial to viscous forces. In straight, smooth tubes, turbulence is probable when the Reynolds number exceeds 2000. The expression shows that turbulence is most likely to occur when the velocity of flow is high and the tube diameter is large (for a given velocity). Note also that a low-density gas like helium tends to produce less turbulence for a given flow rate.

In such a complicated system of tubes as the bronchial tree (*see* Fig. 1–4) with its many branches, changes in caliber, and irregular wall surfaces, the application of the above principles is difficult. In practice, for laminar flow to occur, the entrance conditions of the tube are critical. If eddy formation occurs upstream at a branch point, this disturbance is carried downstream some distance before it disappears. Therefore, in a rapidly branching system like the lung, fully developed laminar flow (Fig. 4–7A) probably only occurs in the very small airways where the Reynolds numbers are very low (approximately 1

in terminal bronchioles during resting breathing). In most of the bronchial tree, flow is transitional (B), while true turbulence may occur in the trachea, especially on exercise when flow velocities are high. In general, driving pressure is determined by both the flow rate and its square: $P = K_1\dot{V} + K_2\dot{V}^2$.

Convection and Diffusion in Airways

The previous section and Figure 4–7 describe the principles of convective flow which occurs in most of the airways. However, deep in the airways in the vicinity of the terminal bronchioles, another mechanism of gas transport begins to become important, and in the alveolar region this mechanism is dominant. This process is diffusion within the airways. It is caused by the random movement of molecules of gas which continually bounce off each other. The reason why diffusion becomes important in the periphery of the airway system can be seen from **FIGURE 4–8.** This shows a plot of the total cross-sectional area of each airway generation, using the idealization of the human airways according to Weibel's model (*see* Fig. 1–5). To derive Figure 4–8, first the cross-sectional area of the trachea (generation 0) is measured, then the cross-sectional areas of the right and left main bronchi (generation 1) are added together, and so on for the subsequent airway generations. There is little difference in total cross-sectional area down to about generation 10, but after about generation 16, which represents the terminal bronchioles, the cross-sectional area increases extremely rapidly.

Because the volume flow through each generation is the same, this very large cross-sectional area means that the forward velocity of the gas is greatly reduced in the very small airways. In fact, in the most peripheral generations, the forward velocity by convective flow becomes so small that diffusion takes over as the dominant mechanism of gas transport. The rate of diffusion of gas molecules within the last few generations of airways is so rapid, and the distances to be covered are so short (a few millimeters), that differences in concentration are virtually abolished within a second.

This change from predominantly convective flow to diffusive transport has important consequences. One is that inhaled dust tends to be deposited in the region of the terminal and

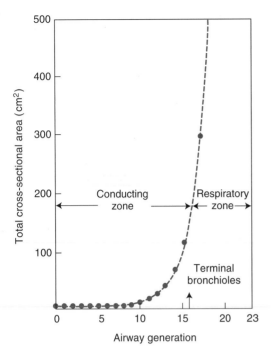

FIGURE 4–8. Diagram to show the extremely rapid increase in total cross-sectional area of the airways in the respiratory zone (compare with Fig. 1-5). As a result, the forward velocity of the gas during inspiration becomes very small in the region of the respiratory bronchioles, and gaseous diffusion becomes the chief mode of ventilation beyond this.

respiratory bronchioles. The reason is that the dust particles, although small, are orders of magnitude more massive than the gas molecules. As a result, their diffusion rates are very small. Consequently, they are not able to diffuse into the most peripheral generations of the airways, and they tend to settle out in the region of the terminal and respiratory bronchioles. This will be discussed further in Chapter 8 (*see* Fig. 8–5).

Measurement of Airway Resistance

Airway resistance is the pressure difference between the alveoli and the mouth divided by the flow rate (Fig. 4–7). Mouth pressure is easily measured with a manometer, and flow rate with a flowmeter. Alveolar pressure is more difficult to obtain, but it can be deduced from measurements made in a body plethysmograph (*see* Fig. 3–8). The subject breathes in and out rapidly, and the pressure in the box is measured. At the

onset of inspiration, the pressure in the alveoli falls as the alveolar gas is slightly expanded. The result is that the gas in the box is slightly compressed and the change of volume in the box (and the lung) can be calculated. If lung volume is known, this change in volume can be converted into alveolar pressure using Boyle's law.

Pressures During the Breathing Cycle

To fully understand the functional consequences of the narrowing of Debra's airways, we need to analyze the pressures in the alveolar and intrapleural spaces during breathing. As already discussed in Chapter 3, a useful measure of intrapleural pressure can be obtained from a balloon catheter in the esophagus.

FIGURE 4–9 shows typical changes in a normal subject. Panel *A* shows that lung volume increases during inspiration and decreases during expiration. Panel *C* shows the corresponding flow rate, with flow increasing during inspiration and then falling to zero at the end of inspiration before it reverses. Panel *D* shows that alveolar pressure is closely related to flow rate. Indeed, because mouth pressure is zero, if airway resistance were constant during the breathing cycle, the changes in alveolar pressure would accurately reflect those of flow.

The only challenging panel in Figure 4–9 is *B*. Intrapleural pressure falls during inspiration, partly because of the increased elastic recoil of the lung (compare with Fig. 3–9). This would take intrapleural pressure along the broken line ABC. In fact, if lung compliance is constant during the breath, the shape of the curve ABC would be identical to the volume changes in panel A. However, there is an additional reason why intrapleural pressure falls during inspiration. This is the reduction in alveolar pressure (panel D) which is necessary for flow to occur. Therefore in panel B, intrapleural pressure actually falls along the solid line AB'C. The vertical distance between the two lines ABC and AB'C reflects the alveolar pressure at any instant, as shown in panel C. As an equation of pressures, (mouth − intrapleural) = (mouth − alveolar) + (alveolar − intrapleural).

Because Debra's airways are narrowed (Fig. 4–1B), airway resistance is greatly increased. The result is that with normal flow rates, the swings in alveolar pressure will be much greater, and intrapleural pressure will also have much larger deflections when flow is occurring. In fact, even during resting expiration, intrapleural pressure may exceed atmospheric pressure.

Chief Site of Airway Resistance

As the airways penetrate toward the periphery of the lung, they become more numerous but much narrower (*see* Figs. 1–4 and 1–5). Based on Poiseuille's equation with its (radius)^4 term, it would be natural to think that the major part of the resistance lies in the very narrow airways. Indeed, this was thought to be the case for many years. However, it has now been shown by direct measurements of the pressure drop along the bronchial tree that the major site of resistance is in the medium-sized bronchi and that the very small bronchioles contribute relatively little resistance. **FIGURE 4–10** shows that most of the resistance occurs in the airways up to about the seventh generation. Less than 20% of the resistance can be attributed to airways less than 2 mm in diameter. The reason for this apparent paradox is the prodigious number of small airways so that although each individual airway has a high resistance, the very large number in parallel have a low resistance.

The fact that the peripheral airways contribute so little resistance is important in the detection of early chronic obstructive pulmonary disease. It is likely that the earliest changes in chronic bronchitis occur in the region of the terminal bronchioles where, as was discussed earlier, much of the pollutant dust settles (*see* Fig. 8–5). However, because these small airways constitute a "silent zone," it is probable that considerable small airway disease can be present before the usual measurements of airway resistance can pick up an abnormality.

In Debra's lung during an asthma attack, most of the airways are narrowed as a result of all the factors shown in Figure 4–1B, and airway resistance is probably increased in all generations of the airways down to the terminal bronchioles.

Factors Determining Airway Resistance

Bronchial Smooth Muscle

All but the smallest peripheral airways have smooth muscle in their walls (Fig. 4–1). Contraction of this muscle narrows the airways and increases their resistance. This may occur re-

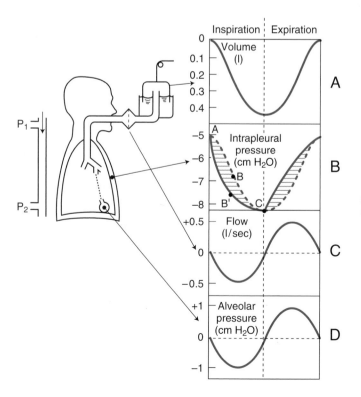

FIGURE 4–9. Volumes, flows, and pressures during the breathing cycle in the normal lung. (See text for details.)

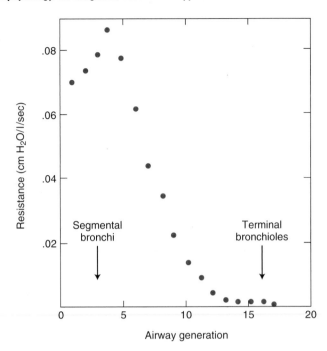

FIGURE 4–10. Location of the chief site of airway resistance. The intermediate-sized bronchi contribute most of the resistance and relatively little is located in the very small airways.

flexly through the stimulation of receptors in the trachea and large bronchi by irritants such as cigarette smoke. Motor innervation is by the vagus nerve. Irritant receptors in the airways were briefly discussed in Chapter 2.

The resting tone (degree of contraction) of the airway smooth muscle is under the control of the autonomic nervous system. This is discussed in more detail later in this chapter in connection with bronchoactive drugs. Stimulation of β_2-adrenergic receptors causes bronchodilatation, as do epinephrine and norepinephrine and drugs such as isoproterenol. Parasympathetic activity causes bronchoconstriction, as does acetylcholine. In addition, a fall of P_{CO_2} in alveolar gas causes an increase in airway resistance, apparently as a result of a direct action on bronchiolar smooth muscle.

Lung Volume

This has an important effect on airway resistance. Like the extra-alveolar blood vessels (*see* Fig. 1–13), the bronchi are supported by the radial traction of the surrounding lung tissue, and their caliber is increased as the lung expands. **FIGURE 4–11** shows that as lung volume is reduced, airway resistance rises rapidly. If the

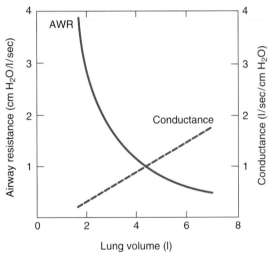

FIGURE 4–11. Effect of lung volume on airway resistance (*AWR*). If the reciprocal of airway resistance or conductance is plotted, the graph is nearly a straight line.

reciprocal of resistance (conductance) is plotted against lung volume, an approximately linear relationship is obtained with conductance falling to very low levels at small lung volumes.

At very low lung volumes, the small airways may close completely (*see* Fig. 3–12). As indicated earlier, Debra has increased lung volumes, especially during an asthma attack. The result is that the airway resistance is reduced below what it would be if lung volume was normal. We saw in Chapter 3 that Chuck, who had chronic obstructive pulmonary disease, also breathed at a high lung volume (*see* Table 3–1). Indeed, it probably would be impossible for Chuck to breathe at all at a normal volume because his airways would be closed!

Gas Density and Viscosity

These affect the resistance offered to flow, as discussed earlier. For example, flow resistance increases during a deep dive because the greatly increased pressure raises gas density. Breathing a helium-oxygen mixture is then beneficial because helium is much less dense than nitrogen. The fact that changes in density rather than viscosity have such an influence on resistance is evidence that flow is not purely laminar in the medium-sized airways, where the main site of resistance lies (Fig. 4–10).

Uneven Ventilation Determined From the Single-Breath Nitrogen Test

Suppose a patient takes a single vital capacity inspiration of oxygen and then slowly exhales to residual volume. If we measure the nitrogen concentration at the mouthpiece with a rapid nitrogen analyzer, we record a pattern as shown in **FIGURE 4–12**. Four phases can be recognized. In the first, which is very short, pure oxygen is exhaled from the upper airways and the nitrogen concentration is zero. In the second phase, the nitrogen concentration rises rapidly as the anatomic dead space is washed out by alveolar gas. This phase is also short.

The third phase consists of alveolar gas, and the tracing is almost flat in normal subjects. This is known as the *alveolar plateau*. In patients with uneven ventilation such as Debra, the third phase steadily rises, and the slope is a measure of the inequality of ventilation. It is expressed as the percentage increase in nitrogen concentration per liter of expired volume. In carrying out

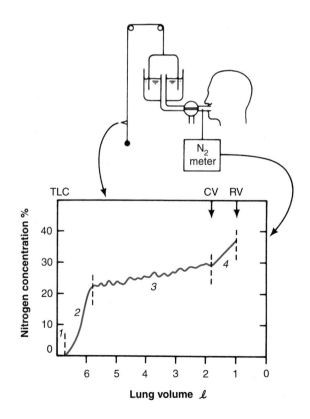

FIGURE 4–12. Single-breath nitrogen test of uneven ventilation. Phase 3 is the alveolar plateau, and the slope of this is a measure of the inequality of ventilation. The onset of phase 4 indicates the closing volume.

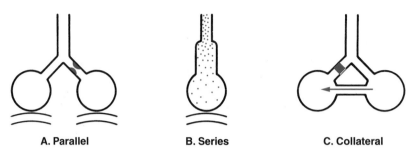

A. Parallel   **B. Series**   **C. Collateral**

FIGURE 4–13. Three mechanisms of uneven ventilation. **A.** Flow to regions behind partly obstructed airways is reduced. **B.** Dilatation of a small airway may result in impaired diffusion along a terminal lung unit. **C.** Lung units behind completely obstructed airways may receive inspired gas from neighboring units.

this test, the expiratory flow rate should be less than $0.5 \, l \cdot sec^{-1}$ to reduce the variability of the results.

The reasons for the rise in concentration in phase 3 are not fully understood. Apparently, some regions of lung are poorly ventilated and therefore receive relatively little of the breath of oxygen. These areas therefore have a relatively high concentration of nitrogen because there is less oxygen to dilute this gas. Also, these poorly ventilated regions tend to empty last.

Three possible mechanisms of uneven ventilation are shown in **FIGURE 4–13**. In A, the region is poorly ventilated because of partial obstruction of its airway and, because of this high resistance, the region empties late. In fact, the rate of emptying of such a region is determined by its time constant, which is given by the product of its airway resistance (R) and compliance (C). The larger the time constant (RC), the longer it takes to empty. This mechanism is known as *parallel inequality* of ventilation.

Figure 4–13B shows a different mechanism, known as *series inequality*. Here there is dilation of peripheral air spaces, causing differences of ventilation *along* the air passages of a lung unit. This type of uneven ventilation may occur in patients with emphysema who have destruction of lung parenchyma (*see* Figs. 3–2B and 3–3B). Under these conditions, the concentration of inspired gas in the most distal airways remains low. Again, these poorly ventilated regions empty last.

Figure 4–13C shows another form of series inequality that occurs when some lung units receive their inspired gas from neighboring units rather than from the large airways. This is known as *collateral ventilation* and appears to be an important process in asthma because, as

Figures 4–5 and 4–6 show, patients with asthma typically have no shunt (completely unventilated but perfused lung) even though some of their airways are completely occluded by mucous plugs. The same mechanism probably occurs in patients with chronic bronchitis (*see* Fig. 3–23).

Closing Volume

Toward the end of the expiration shown in Figure 4–12, the nitrogen concentration rose abruptly, signaling the onset of phase 4. The volume of the onset of phase 4 above residual volume is called the *closing volume*, and the closing volume plus the residual volume is sometimes known as the *closing capacity*. In practice, the onset of phase 4 is obtained by drawing a straight line through the alveolar plateau (phase 3) and noting the last point of departure of the nitrogen tracing from this line. This is difficult to measure in severe lung disease.

The mechanism of the onset of phase 4 is not fully understood, but many researchers believe that it is caused by closure of small airways in the lowest part of the lung. At residual volume just before the single breath of oxygen is taken, the nitrogen concentration is virtually uniform throughout the lung, but the basal alveoli are much smaller than the apical alveoli in the upright subject because of distortion of the lung by its weight (*see* Fig. 3–12). However, at the end of a vital capacity inspiration, all the alveoli are approximately the same size. Therefore, the nitrogen concentration at the apex is diluted much less than that at the base by the breath of oxygen.

During the subsequent expiration, the upper and lower zones empty together and the expired nitrogen concentration is nearly constant (Fig. 4–12). However, as soon as dependent airways begin to close, the higher nitrogen concentration in the upper zones preferentially affects the expired concentration, causing an abrupt rise. Moreover, as airway closure proceeds up the lung, the expired nitrogen progressively increases.

However, recent studies show that in some subjects, the closing volume is the same in the weightlessness of space as in normal gravity. This unexpected finding suggests that compression of dependent lung is not the only mechanism, and it emphasizes how uncertain we are about this topic.

The volume at which airways close is very age-dependent, being as low as 10% of the vital capacity in young subjects but increasing to 40% (that is, approximately the FRC) at about the age of 65 years. There is some evidence that the test is sensitive to small amounts of disease. For example, apparently healthy cigarette smokers sometimes have increased closing volumes when their ventilatory capacity is normal.

□ PATHOGENESIS OF ASTHMA

This is a convenient place to briefly discuss the physiological principles of bronchoactive drugs because of their great importance in the management of asthma. However, an introductory section on the pathogenesis of asthma is neces-sary. Rapid progress is being made in this area, and the following account will no doubt be modified before long.

Two features that appear to be common to all persons with asthma are airway hyperrespon-siveness and airway inflammation. Recent research suggests that the hyperresponsiveness is a consequence of the inflammation, and some investigators believe that airway inflammation is responsible for all the associated features of asthma, including the increased airway respon-siveness, airway edema, hypersecretion of mucus, and inflammatory cell infiltration. However, a fundamental abnormality of airway smooth muscle or regulation of airway tone is possible in some patients.

The trigger for the development of airway inflammation cannot always be identified. It is well recognized in some instances, as in the case of some antigens in persons with allergic asthma **(FIGURE 4–14)**. However, in other types of asthma, such as exercise-induced asthma or asthma following a viral respiratory tract infection, the trigger is not recognized. Atmospheric pollutants, especially submicronic particles in automobile exhaust gases, may also play a role.

A single inflammatory cell type or inflammatory mediator does not appear to be responsible for all the manifestations of asthma. Eosinophils, mast cells, neutrophils, macrophages, and basophils have all been implicated. There is also evidence that noninflammatory cells, including

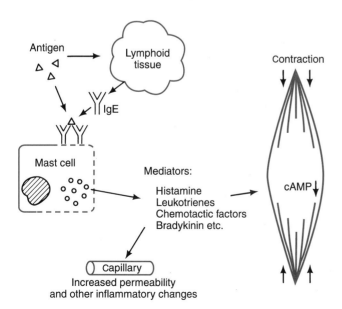

FIGURE 4–14. Some pathogenic changes in allergic asthma. (See text for details.)

airway epithelial cells and neural cells, especially those of peptidergic nerves, contribute to the inflammation. Some investigators believe that eosinophils play a central effective role in most cases of asthma. There is also evidence that lymphocytes, especially T cells, are implicated, both because they respond to specific antigens and because they play a role as a modulator of inflammatory cell function.

Many inflammatory mediators have been identified in asthma. Cytokines are probably important, particularly those associated with Th-2, helper T-cell activation. These cytokines include granulocyte-macrophage colony-stimulating factor, interleukin-3 (IL-3), IL-4, and IL-5. It is believed that these cytokines are at least partly responsible for modulating inflammatory and immune cell function, and for supporting the inflammatory response in the airway. Other inflammatory mediators that probably play a role, particularly in acute bronchoconstriction, include arachidonic acid metabolites, such as leukotrienes and prostaglandins, platelet-activating factor (PAF), neuropeptides, reactive oxygen species, kinins, histamine, and adenosine.

Asthma also has a genetic component. Population studies show that it is a complex genetic disorder with both environmental and genetic components.

☐ BRONCHOACTIVE DRUGS

Drugs that reverse or prevent bronchoconstriction have a major role in the management of asthma. They are also useful in those patients with chronic bronchitis who have some reversible airway obstruction. The principles, rather than details, of their use will be considered briefly.

β-Adrenergic Agonists

β-Adrenergic receptors are of two types. β_1 receptors exist in the heart and elsewhere, and their stimulation increases heart rate and the force of contraction of cardiac muscle. Stimulation of β_2 receptors relaxes smooth muscle in the bronchi, blood vessels, and uterus. Partially or completely β_2-selective adrenergic agonists have now completely replaced nonselective agonists in the treatment of asthma. Available drugs include albuterol, terbutaline, and pirbuterol. These agents have an intermediate duration of action. Long-acting agents, such as salmeterol,

are also available but should only be used on a regular schedule, not for acute relief of symptoms. All these drugs bind to β_2 receptors in the lungs and directly relax airway smooth muscle by increasing the activity of adenyl cyclase. This in turn raises the concentration of intracellular cAMP which is reduced in an asthma attack (Fig. 4–14). These drugs also have effects on airway edema and airway inflammation. Their anti-inflammatory effects are mediated by direct inhibition of inflammatory cell function via binding to β_2 receptors on the cell surface.

These drugs are delivered by aerosol, preferably using a metered-dose inhaler, or a nebulizer. In the past, there has been concern about possible tachyphylaxis (reduced efficacy with frequent use), particularly in the drug's ability to reverse induced bronchoconstriction when used regularly. However, this is now less of an issue.

Corticosteroids

These appear to have two separate functions: they inhibit the inflammatory/immune response, and they enhance β receptor expression or function. Inhaled corticosteroids are now increasingly used in the management of asthma. Some physicians argue that all patients with asthma benefit from inhaled corticosteroids. However, other physicians feel that patients who experience symptoms less than three times a week, and whose conditions are easily controlled with intermittent β_2 agonists, do not require corticosteroids. A wide variety of inhaled corticosteroids are now currently available and, when used as directed, result in minimal systemic absorption of corticosteroids with almost no serious side effects.

Methylxanthines

The mechanism of action of these, including theophylline and aminophylline, is uncertain. They have modest anti-inflammatory properties and are also bronchodilators, although they are much less potent than β_2 agonists. The therapeutic dose is close to the toxic dose, but they are still useful in the management of chronic asthma. Measurement of blood levels is an aid to developing the correct dose.

Anticholinergics

There is evidence that the parasympathetic nervous system may play a part in the asthma reaction. However, anticholinergics have only a modest bronchodilating effect and only in a subset of patients with asthma. By contrast, patients with chronic obstructive pulmonary disease with reversible bronchoconstriction respond more consistently, and anticholinergics are useful here.

Cromolyn and Nedocromil

Although these two drugs are structurally unrelated, they apparently have similar mechanisms of action. They were originally thought to be mast cell stabilizers (Fig. 4–14), but it is now recognized that they have broad-ranging effects. They are not direct bronchodilators but presumably work by blocking airway inflammation.

New Therapies

Leukotriene receptor antagonists and 5-lipoxygenase inhibitors are available, but their role in clinical asthma therapy is still unclear. There is some evidence that receptor antagonists are valuable in severe, persistent asthma. There is also ongoing research on other inhibitors.

Questions   For each question, choose the one best answer.
(For answers, see p. 150.)

1. All of the following pathological changes occur in the airways in asthma EXCEPT:
   A. Edema of the bronchial wall
   B. Hypertrophy of bronchial mucous glands
   C. Hypertrophy of smooth muscle
   D. Abnormal mucus
   E. Destruction of small airways

2. When a bronchodilator is administered to a patient with asthma during an attack, all of the following typically increase EXCEPT:
   A. FEV_1
   B. FEV/FVC%
   C. FVC
   D. $FEF_{25-75\%}$
   E. FRC

3. Concerning airflow in the lung:
   A. The higher the Reynolds number, the less likely is turbulence to occur.
   B. For inspiration to occur, mouth pressure must be less than alveolar pressure.
   C. In pure laminar flow, halving the radius of the airway increases its resistance eightfold.
   D. In pure laminar flow, doubling the length of the airway increases its resistance fourfold.
   E. Flow is more likely to be turbulent in small airways than in the trachea.

4. A normal subject makes an inspiratory effort against a closed airway. All of the following are true EXCEPT:
   A. Tension in the diaphragm increases.
   B. The external intercostal muscles become active.
   C. Intrapleural pressure falls.
   D. Alveolar pressure falls more than intrapleural pressure.
   E. Pressure inside the pulmonary capillaries falls.

5. Which of the following statements about normal expiration during resting conditions is FALSE?
   A. Alveolar pressure is greater than atmospheric pressure.
   B. Flow velocity of the gas in the large airways exceeds that in the terminal bronchioles.
   C. Diaphragm moves headward.
   D. Intrapleural pressure gradually falls (becomes more negative).
   E. Normal expiration is generated by the elastic forces of the lung.

6. All of the following factors increase pulmonary airway resistance EXCEPT:
   A. Reducing lung volume below FRC
   B. Increased sympathetic stimulation of airway smooth muscle
   C. Diving to a great depth
   D. Inhaling cigarette smoke
   E. Breathing a mixture of 21% O_2 and 79% sulfur hexafluoride (molecular weight 146)

7. Features of the pathogenesis of asthma include all of the following EXCEPT:
   A. Airway inflammation
   B. Airway hyperresponsiveness
   C. Hypersecretion of mucus
   D. Liberation of cytokines
   E. Bronchial artery thrombosis

8. The following statements about the use of β-adrenergic agonists in asthma are true EXCEPT:
   A. β_2-selective agonists are preferred to β_1 agonists.
   B. They relax airway smooth muscle by raising the concentration of adenyl cyclase.
   C. They reduce the concentration of intracellular cAMP.
   D. They reduce airway inflammation.
   E. They reduce airway edema.

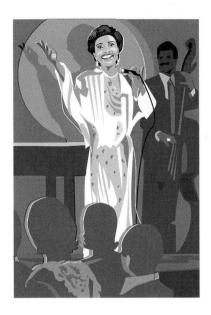

Chapter 5

Diffuse Interstitial Pulmonary Fibrosis

☐ Elena is a 40-year-old nightclub singer whose chief complaints are increasing shortness of breath and fatigue over the past 5 years. On examination, she had rapid, shallow breathing and was unable to make a large inspiration. A chest radiograph showed contracted lungs with a reticular pattern suggesting interstitial fibrosis, and this diagnosis was confirmed by a lung biopsy. We review the normal structure of the alveoli and the pathological changes of interstitial fibrosis. The consequences of reduced lung compliance are discussed, as is the impairment of diffusion caused by the thickened blood-gas barrier.

☐ CLINICAL FINDINGS

History

Elena is a 40-year-old blues singer whose chief complaints are dyspnea and fatigue. She was well until about 5 years ago, when she began to notice increasing shortness of breath which was particularly obvious when she was singing or climbing stairs. At the same time, she began to feel unusually fatigued and experienced some weight loss. She also developed an irritating, unproductive cough. There was no chest pain, the patient was a nonsmoker, and there was no family history of lung disease. She was not apparently exposed to dusts or other substances that are toxic to the lung.

Physical Examination

The patient looked rather drawn, and there was rapid, shallow breathing, frequency 25 per min. There was no cyanosis at rest. However, finger "clubbing" was present, that is, there was an increase in tissue mass at the base of the nails with the result that the fingers approached the shape of drumsticks. Examination of the chest showed a poor inspiratory movement when the patient was asked to take a full inspiration. On auscultation, fine inspiratory crepitations (crackles) could be heard over both lungs. The cardiovascular system was normal except for a loud pulmonary second sound. There was no neck vein engorgement, palpable liver, or dependent edema. The results of examinations of other systems were normal.

Investigations

Blood studies showed a normal hemoglobin and cell counts. A chest radiograph showed a small, contracted lung and rib cage with raised diaphragms (FIGURE 5–1). The original film showed a fine reticular pattern throughout both lungs with areas of more pronounced shadowing.

Exercise Test

The patient walked on a treadmill in the pulmonary function laboratory. Her maximal oxygen consumption was $2.2 \, l \cdot min^{-1}$ which was very low. She could not exercise at a higher work rate because of shortness of breath. Her blood gases on exercise are shown in TABLE 5–1.

Lung Biopsy

A biopsy was done during bronchoscopy to come to a definitive diagnosis. The specimen (FIGURE 5–2) showed marked thickening of the alveolar walls as a result of extensive collagen deposition. There was also cellular infiltration. Many of the capillaries were obliterated by fibrous tissue.

Diagnosis

Diffuse interstitial pulmonary fibrosis of unknown cause.

Treatment and Progress

The patient was treated with the corticosteroid, prednisone, and this resulted in marked im-

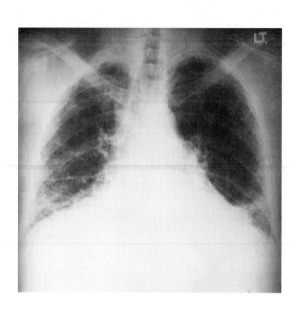

FIGURE 5–1. Chest radiograph of a patient with diffuse interstitial pulmonary fibrosis. Note the small contracted lung and rib cage as well as the raised diaphragms (compare with normal appearance of lung in Fig. 3-1). The original film showed a fine reticular pattern in the lung fields, but this does not reproduce well.

TABLE 5–1
Pulmonary Function Tests

Lung Volumes and Compliance		Observed	Predicted
VC (liters)		3.1	4.0
FRC (liters)		2.3	3.2
TLC (liters)		4.5	5.6
Compliance ($l \cdot cm\ H_2O^{-1}$)		0.11	0.20
Forced Expiration			
FEV_1 (liters)		2.8	3.2
FVC (liters)		3.1	4.0
FEV/FVC%		90	81
$FEF_{25-75\%}$ ($l \cdot sec^{-1}$)		3.7	3.5
Arterial Blood Gases			
P_{O_2} (mm Hg)	Rest	61	>90
	Exercise	46	>90
P_{CO_2} (mm Hg)	Rest	35	40
	Exercise	35	40
pH	Rest	7.43	7.40
	Exercise	7.43	7.40
Diffusing Capacity for CO			
($ml \cdot min^{-1} \cdot mm\ Hg^{-1}$)		11	25

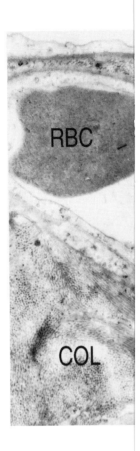

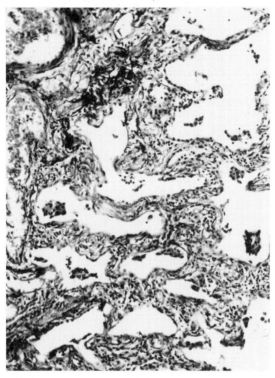

FIGURE 5–2. Biopsy specimen of lung from a patient with diffuse interstitial pulmonary fibrosis. Note the marked thickening of the alveolar walls and loss of pulmonary capillaries.

tion and small lung volumes. However, both types of disease are severely disabling, with greatly altered mechanical properties of the lung and marked impairment of gas exchange.

Interstitial lung disease primarily affects the parenchyma or alveolar tissue of the lung. Therefore let's start by looking at the structure of the normal alveoli.

Structure of the Normal Alveolar Wall

This is a good time to review Figure 1–7, which shows an electron micrograph of a capillary in a normal alveolar wall. Recall that the thin side of the blood-gas barrier is typically less than 0.3 μm thick and contains three layers: alveolar epithelium, interstitium, and capillary endothelium.

Type I Epithelial Cell

This is the chief structural cell of the alveolar wall. Its shape is something like a fried egg because it has a central nucleus and long protoplasmic extensions that pave almost the whole alveolar surface (see Fig. 1–7). The main function of this cell is mechanical support. It rarely divides and is not metabolically active. When type I cells are injured, they cannot repair themselves, and they are replaced by type II epithelial cells.

Type II Epithelial Cell

This is a nearly globular cell (**FIGURE 5–3**) and so it is easily distinguished from a type I cell. It provides little structural support for the alveolar wall, but is metabolically very active. The electron micrograph shows the lamellated bodies (*LB*) that contain phospholipid. This is eventually extruded into the alveolar space to form surfactant, which will be discussed in Chapter 6. After injury to the alveolar wall, these cells rapidly divide to line the surface and are later transformed into type I epithelial cells.

Other Cells

These include alveolar macrophages. This scavenger cell roams around the alveolar wall and engulfs foreign particles and bacteria by phagocytosis. The cell contains lysozymes that digest engulfed foreign matter. Figure 1–7 also shows a

provement. Her dyspnea improved considerably, and the patient was able to resume most of her normal activities, including singing. The chest radiograph showed resolution of most of the reticular pattern in the lung, although the lungs remained small.

☐ NORMAL HISTOLOGY AND PATHOLOGY

Elena shows many of the common features of diffuse interstitial pulmonary fibrosis, one of the group of interstitial lung diseases. A discussion of her clinical findings, investigations, pathology, and pathophysiology can be very instructive. In some ways, the functional abnormalities in her disease are a mirror image of what we saw in Chuck, who had chronic obstructive pulmonary disease, and Debra, who had asthma. These last two patients had obstructive lung disease, characterized by airway obstruction and large lung volumes. By contrast, Elena has restrictive lung disease, with essentially no airway obstruc-

trauma, infection, or
interstitial pulmonary
many forms of injury,
to determine what the
as a scar on the arm is
so interstitial pulmona
stiff and greatly reduce

Following this br
structural changes in
discuss the functiona
sulted in Elena's clini
monary function tests.

☐ PHYSIOLOGY PATHOPHYSIC

Clinical Findings

History

One of Elena's chief
and a major cause of
compliant lung which
The result is that it
increase her ventilatio
work capacity was th
only 2.2 l · min⁻¹). Th

fibroblast (*FB*), which syr
elastin. In diffuse interstit
large amounts of collager
interstitium of the alveola

Interstitium of the Al

This occupies the space
epithelium and capillary e
1–7 shows, it is often th
capillary, where it consi:
basement membranes of
and capillary endothelial l
the blood-gas barrier is vu
failure because it is so
mechanical strength of
blood-gas barrier comes
apparently predominantl
collagen which is a major

On the other side
interstitium is usually wio
of type I collagen (COL
as fibroblasts and pericy
chiefly concerned with fl
capillary wall (*see* Chapte
side is responsible for mc

FIGURE 5–3. Electron mi
graph of a type II alve
epithelial cell. Note the lar
lated bodies (*LB*), large
cleus, and microvilli (*arro*
and the cytoplasm which
rich in organelles. The *inse*
top right is a scanning e
tron micrograph showing
surface view of a type II
with its characteristic distr
tion of microvilli.

and other shadowing in the lung fields were caused by fibrosis of the alveolar walls. Sometimes the radiograph shows a typical honeycomb appearance caused by dilated small airways as referred to above.

Pulmonary Function Tests

Lung Volumes and Compliance

All lung volumes were reduced because the fibrosis of the alveolar wall made Elena's lungs stiff and difficult to expand (Table 5–1). As a consequence of the fibrosis there was a greatly reduced compliance. Figure 4–4 showed a typical pressure-volume curve of the lung in interstitial fibrosis. Note that (1) it is much flatter than normal and (2) there is a very high transpulmonary pressure of over 40 cm H_2O at total lung capacity. This very high pressure is developed because the lungs are extremely stiff and resist expansion, and the outwardly expanding chest wall can generate a very large (negative) pressure at low volumes. By contrast, Figure 4–4 shows that the transpulmonary pressure at total lung capacity in emphysema is abnormally small, as would be the case in Chuck.

The small lungs of patients with interstitial pulmonary fibrosis, and the large lungs of patients with emphysema (*see* Figs. 3–1B and 4–4), are related to the different lung compliances in the two conditions. However, strictly speaking, the volumes are determined by the interactions between the recoil forces of the lung and chest wall. This is a convenient place to describe these briefly. This topic can be confusing at first, because while it is easy to see intuitively that the lung is recoiling inward, it is less obvious that the chest wall is recoiling outward.

First, we can appreciate the interactions between the lung and chest wall by looking at the simple example of a pneumothorax (**FIGURE 5–5**). This shows that the normal pressure outside the lung in the intrapleural space is

subatmospheric, just as it is in the jar of Figure 3–9. When air is introduced into the intrapleural space, either because a bleb on the surface of the lung ruptures or because of a penetrating injury to the chest wall, the pressure in the space becomes atmospheric. As a result, the lung recoils inward and the chest wall springs out. This behavior emphasizes that under normal equilibrium conditions, the chest wall is pulled inward while the lung is pulled outward, the two pulls balancing each other.

However, to understand these interactions fully we need to discuss the so-called *relaxation pressure-volume curves* of the lung and chest wall (**FIGURE 5–6**). To make these measurements, the subject inspires from, or expires into, a spirometer to a designated lung volume. The airway is then occluded with a tap (drawing in Fig. 5–6), and the subject relaxes the respiratory muscles while the airway pressure is measured ("relaxation pressure"). Incidentally, this is difficult for an untrained subject to do.

Figure 5–6 shows that at functional residual capacity (FRC), the relaxation pressure of the lung plus chest wall is atmospheric. Indeed, FRC is the equilibrium volume when the elastic recoil of the lung is exactly balanced by the normal tendency for the chest wall to spring out. At volumes above FRC, the relaxation pressure is positive, and at smaller volumes, the pressure is subatmospheric.

Figure 5–6 also shows the curve for the lung alone. This is similar to the curve shown in Figure 3–9, except that for clarity no hysteresis is indicated, and the pressures are positive instead of negative. They are the pressures that would be found from the experiment of Figure 3–9 if, after the lung had reached a certain volume, the line to the spirometer was clamped, the jar opened to the atmosphere (so that the lung relaxed against the closed airway), and the airway pressure measured. At zero pressure the lung is at its *minimal volume*, which is below residual volume.

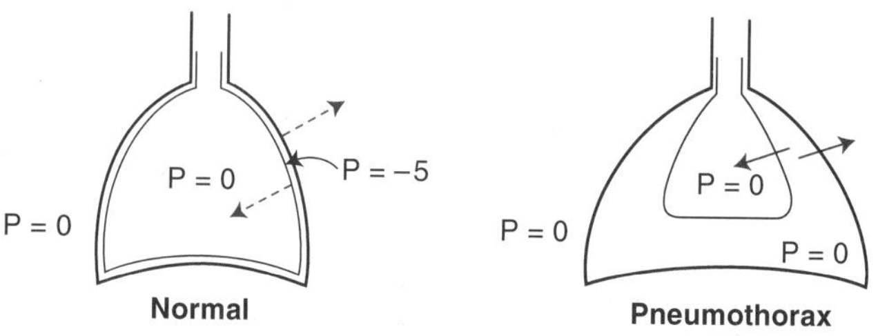

FIGURE 5–5. The tendency of the lung to recoil to its deflated volume is balanced by the tendency of the chest cage to bow out. As a result, the intrapleural pressure is subatmospheric. Pneumothorax allows the lung to collapse and the thorax to spring out.

P = 0   P = 0   P = −5

Normal

P = 0   P = 0   P = 0

Pneumothorax

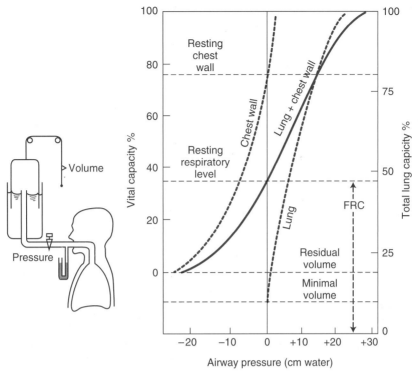

FIGURE 5–6. Relaxation pressure-volume curve of the lung and chest wall. The subject inspires (or expires) to a predetermined volume from the spirometer, the tap is closed, and he or she then relaxes the respiratory muscles. Note that the curve for lung plus chest wall can be explained by the addition of the individual lung and chest wall curves.

The third curve is for the chest wall only. We can imagine this being measured on a subject with a normal chest wall and no lung! At FRC, the relaxation pressure is negative (subatmospheric). In other words, at this volume the chest cage is tending to spring out. It is not until the volume is increased to about 75% of the vital capacity that the relaxation pressure is atmospheric, that is the chest wall has found its equilibrium position. At every volume, the relaxation pressure of the lung plus chest wall is the sum of the pressures for the lung and the chest wall measured separately.

Applying this information to our two patients, Chuck (chronic obstructive pulmonary disease) and Elena (diffuse interstitial pulmonary fibrosis), it is likely that the relaxation pressure-volume curve of the chest wall is normal in both cases, at least in the early stages of disease. Therefore, the reduced elastic recoil of the lung in the case of Chuck means that the FRC volume must be increased. By contrast, the increased elastic recoil and therefore reduced compliance of the lung in the case of Elena means that her FRC must be reduced.

Forced Expiration

Table 5–1 shows that Elena's forced vital capacity (FVC) was decreased, as would be expected from her greatly reduced lung compliance. In other words, her respiratory muscles were just not able to expand her lung to normal volumes. However, her FEV/FVC% was actually higher than normal. In fact, the pattern of her forced expiration was that depicted in Figure 3–13C. This shows that although the total volume exhaled was reduced, expiration was very rapid. This is confirmed by the abnormally high forced expiratory flow (FEF$_{25-75\%}$).

Additional information can be obtained from a flow-volume curve, and a typical curve for restrictive lung disease was shown in Figure 4–3B. Note first that all lung volumes are reduced because of the low compliance. However, the descending portion of the flow-volume curve shows that flow rates in relation to lung volume are high, and in fact exceed the flow rates (for a given lung volume) in the normal subject. What is the reason for this?

Recall that a normal subject develops dynamic compression of the airways during a forced expiration (*see* Fig. 3–16). This occurs to a much greater extent in a patient like Chuck for the reasons described in Chapter 3. In fact, Chuck may develop dynamic compression of his airways even during a normal resting expiration. One of the reasons for this is depicted in **FIGURE 5–7**, which shows that the airways of the emphysematous lung have lost the normal radial traction given by the surrounding parenchyma because of breakdown of the alveolar walls. By contrast, the fibrotic lung of Elena has its airways pulled open to an abnormally large extent by the contracted fibrous tissue in the alveolar walls, with the result that airway caliber is large when related to lung volume. Therefore, dynamic compression of the airways during a forced expiration is much less likely to occur. A pathological correlate of this is the honeycomb appearance sometimes seen in the chest radiograph which is caused by dilated terminal and respiratory bronchioles surrounded by thickened scar tissue. However, this is not obvious in Figure 5–1.

Arterial Blood Gases

Elena's arterial P_{O_2} was reduced (Table 5–1), and the major mechanism is ventilation-perfusion inequality as discussed in the case of Chuck. Basically the same mechanism applies to Debra's lung. As Figures 5–2 and 5–4 show, there is massive derangement of the normal architecture of the lung at the alveolar level, and it is therefore impossible for ventilation and blood flow to be matched properly. Areas of fibrosis reduce the expansion and therefore ventilation

of some parts of the lung. In addition many capillaries are destroyed by the fibrotic process with the result that regional blood flow is reduced. These two patients highlight the fact that ventilation-perfusion inequality is by far the most common cause of hypoxemia in lung disease.

However, there is an additional reason why the arterial P_{O_2} may be reduced in Elena. This is impairment of diffusion of gas across the blood-gas barrier because this is thickened (Figs. 5–2 and 5–4). Although this subject was introduced in Chapter 1 (*see* Figs. 1–7 to 1–9), we now have an opportunity to look at it in more depth.

Diffusion Across the Blood-Gas Barrier

Fick's law describing the diffusion of gases through a tissue sheet was introduced in Chapter 1 (*see* Fig. 1–8). Now let's look at the uptake of gases along the pulmonary capillary more closely.

Diffusion and Perfusion Limitations

Suppose blood enters a pulmonary capillary of an alveolus which contains a foreign gas such as carbon monoxide or nitrous oxide. How rapidly will the partial pressure in the blood rise? **FIGURE 5–8** shows the time courses as a red blood cell moves through the capillary, a process which we have seen takes about 0.75 sec under resting conditions. First look at carbon monoxide (CO). When a red cell enters the capillary, CO moves rapidly across the extremely thin blood-gas barrier from the alveolar gas into the cell. As a result, the content of CO in the cell rises. However, because of the tight bond that forms between CO and hemoglobin within the cell, a large amount of CO can be taken up by

FIGURE 5–7. Airway caliber in normal lung, emphysema, and interstitial fibrosis. In emphysema, the airways tend to collapse because of the loss of radial traction. By contrast, in fibrosis, radial traction may be excessive, with the result that airway caliber is large when related to lung volume.

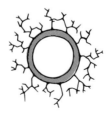
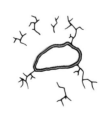
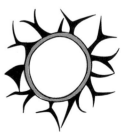

Normal   **Emphysema**   **Fibrosis**

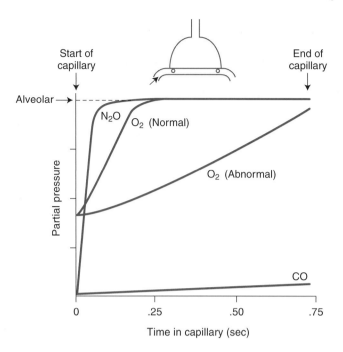

FIGURE 5–8. Uptake of carbon monoxide (CO), nitrous oxide (N₂O), and O₂ along the pulmonary capillary. Note that the blood partial pressure of nitrous oxide virtually reaches that of alveolar gas very early in the capillary so that the transfer of this gas is perfusion limited. By contrast, the partial pressure of carbon monoxide in the blood is almost unchanged so that its transfer is diffusion limited. O₂ transfer can be perfusion limited or partly diffusion limited, depending on the conditions (compare with Fig. 1-9).

the cell with almost no increase in partial pressure. Therefore, as the cell moves through the capillary, the CO partial pressure in the blood hardly changes, so that no appreciable back pressure develops, and the gas continues to move rapidly across the alveolar wall. It is clear therefore that the amount of CO that gets into the blood is limited by the diffusion properties of the blood-gas barrier and not by the amount of blood available. The transfer of CO is therefore said to be *diffusion limited*.

Contrast the time course of nitrous oxide (N₂O). When this gas moves across the alveolar wall into the blood, no combination with hemoglobin takes place. As a result, the blood has nothing like the avidity for nitrous oxide that it has for CO, and the partial pressure in the blood rises rapidly. Indeed, Figure 5–8 shows that the partial pressure of nitrous oxide in the blood has virtually reached that of the alveolar gas by the time the red cell is only one-tenth of the way along the capillary. After this point, almost no nitrous oxide is transferred. Thus, the amount of this gas taken up by the blood depends entirely on the amount of available blood flow, and not at all on the diffusion properties of the blood-gas barrier. The transfer of nitrous oxide is therefore *perfusion-limited*.

What of O₂? As Figure 5–8 shows, its time course lies between those of CO and nitrous oxide. O₂ combines with hemoglobin (unlike nitrous oxide), but with nothing like the avidity of CO. In other words, the rise in partial pressure when O₂ enters a red cell is much greater than is the case for the same number of molecules of CO. Figure 5–8 shows that under typical resting conditions, the capillary P_{O_2} virtually reaches that of alveolar gas when the red cell is about one-third of the way along the capillary. Under these conditions, O₂ transfer is perfusion-limited, like nitrous oxide. However, in a patient like Elena in whom the diffusion properties of the lung are impaired because of the thickening of the blood-gas barrier (Figs. 5–2 and 5–4), the P_{O_2} of the blood may not reach the alveolar value by the end of the capillary, and now there is some diffusion-limitation as well. This is particularly likely to be the case on exercise when the time spent by the blood in the capillary is greatly reduced (*see* Fig. 1–9).

A more detailed analysis shows that whether a gas is diffusion-limited or not depends essentially on its solubility in the blood-gas barrier compared with its "solubility" in blood (actually, the slope of the dissociation curve; *see* Fig. 1–14). For a gas like CO, these are very different, whereas for a gas like nitrous oxide they are the same. An analogy is the rate at which sheep can enter a field through a gate. If the gate is narrow but the field is large, the number of sheep that can enter in a given time is limited by the size of the gate. However, if both the gate and the field are small (or both are big), the number of sheep is limited by the size of the field.

We have seen that both thickening of the blood-gas barrier and exercise can potentially result in diffusion limitation of oxygen transfer. Another cause is alveolar hypoxia. As we saw in Chapter 2, Bill's alveolar P_{O_2} at high altitude was reduced from the normal value of 100 to 75. This means that the driving pressure for oxygen diffusion across the blood-gas barrier is reduced. In addition, however, at very high altitude, loading of O_2 by the pulmonary capillary takes place low on the O_2 dissociation curve (*see* Fig. 1–14) where its slope is very steep. Under these circumstances, O_2 is beginning to behave like CO as far as diffusion is concerned. Therefore, at extreme altitude, Bill is likely to have some diffusion limitation of O_2 transfer at rest, and this will be greatly exaggerated during exercise when the time spent by the blood in the capillary is reduced. Severe exercise at very high altitude is the best example of a situation where diffusion limitation of O_2 transfer is seen in normal subjects.

Measurement of Diffusing Capacity

It is sometimes valuable to know whether the diffusion properties of a lung are abnormal. A good example is Elena, in whom the initial clinical presentation suggested interstitial fibrosis, and a measurement of diffusing capacity would help to confirm the diagnosis. How can we measure the diffusion properties of the lung in a living patient? Clearly, the gas of choice is carbon monoxide because its uptake is so clearly diffusion limited (Fig. 5–8).

Fick's law of diffusion (*see* Fig. 1–8) can be written:

$$\dot{V}\,gas = \frac{A}{T} \cdot D \cdot (P_1 - P_2)$$

where A is the area of the blood-gas barrier, T is its thickness, and D is a diffusion constant.

Now for a complex structure like the blood-gas barrier, it is not possible to measure the area and thickness during life. Instead, the equation is rewritten:

$$\dot{V}\,gas = D_L \cdot (P_1 - P_2)$$

where D_L is called the *diffusing capacity of the lung* and includes the area, thickness, and diffusion properties of the tissue sheet and the gas concerned. Therefore, the diffusing capacity for carbon monoxide is given by:

$$D_L = \frac{\dot{V}_{CO}}{P_1 - P_2}$$

where P_1 and P_2 are the partial pressures of alveolar gas and capillary blood, respectively. However, as we have seen (Fig. 5–8), the partial pressure of CO in capillary blood is extremely small and it can generally be neglected. Therefore:

$$D_L = \frac{\dot{V}_{CO}}{P_{A_{CO}}}$$

or, in words, the diffusing capacity of the lung for CO is the volume of CO transferred in ml per minute per mm Hg of alveolar partial pressure.

For this measurement, Elena took a single inspiration of a dilute mixture of CO in air (about 0.3% CO), held her breath for 10 seconds, and then exhaled. The concentrations of CO in the inspired and expired gas were then measured and the rate of disappearance of CO from the lung was calculated. The CO concentration in the alveolar gas was not constant during the breath-holding period because it was continually absorbed by the blood, but allowance was made for that. Also, a small concentration of helium was added to the inspired gas to give a measurement of lung volume by dilution. Table 5–1 shows that Elena's diffusing capacity for CO measured in this way was only 11 ml · min^{-1} · mm Hg^{-1}, whereas the predicted normal value was 25. This measurement is therefore consistent with the clinical presentation and the lung biopsy results (Fig. 5–2). Indeed, if the measured diffusing capacity had been normal, this would be strong evidence against a diagnosis of interstitial fibrosis.

Reaction Rates With Hemoglobin

So far we have assumed that all the resistance to the movement of O_2 and CO resides in the barrier between blood and gas. However, Figure 1–7 shows that the path length from the alveolar wall to the center of a red blood cell exceeds that in the wall itself, so that some of the diffusion resistance is located within the capillary. In addition, there is another type of resistance to gas transfer that is most conveniently discussed with diffusion, that is, the resistance caused by the finite rate of reaction of O_2 or CO with hemoglobin inside the red cell. These rates can slow the uptake of O_2 or CO in the lung, and the end result is very like the effects of reduced diffusion.

When O_2 (or CO) is added to blood, its combination with hemoglobin is quite fast, being well on the way to completion in 0.2 sec. However, oxygenation occurs so rapidly in the pulmonary capillary (*see* Figs. 1–9 and 5–8) that even this rapid reaction significantly delays the loading of O_2 (or CO) by the red cell. Therefore, the uptake of O_2 (or CO) can be regarded as occurring in two stages: (1) diffusion of O_2 through the blood-gas barrier (including the plasma and red cell interior), and (2) reaction of O_2 with hemoglobin **(FIGURE 5–9)**. In fact, it is possible to sum the two resultant resistances to produce an overall "diffusion" resistance.

The details of how this is done need not concern us, but the complete equation is:

$$\frac{1}{D_L} = \frac{1}{D_M} + \frac{1}{\theta \cdot V_c}$$

where D_L is the diffusing capacity of the lung for carbon monoxide, D_M is the diffusing capacity of the "membrane" (including the plasma), θ is the rate of reaction of O_2 (or CO) with hemoglobin, and V_c is the volume of blood in the pulmonary capillaries. This equation shows that the measured D_L can be lowered not only by a reduction in the diffusion properties of the membrane but also by reductions in θ and V_c. In fact, a fall in V_c, that is the capillary blood volume, is a factor in Elena's reduced diffusing capacity because, as Figure 5–2 shows, many of the pulmonary capillaries have been obliterated by the interstitial fibrosis. Note also that θ for CO can be reduced by giving Elena a high oxygen mixture to breathe, because under these conditions, O_2 competes with CO for the

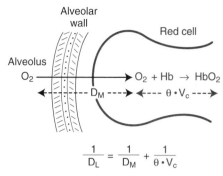

$$\frac{1}{D_L} = \frac{1}{D_M} + \frac{1}{\theta \cdot V_c}$$

FIGURE 5–9. The diffusing capacity of the lung (D_L) is made up of two components: that due to the diffusion process itself, and that attributable to the time taken for O_2 (or CO) to react with hemoglobin. (See text for details.)

hemoglobin and therefore θ for CO is reduced. In fact, it is possible to manipulate the value of θ by changing the alveolar P_{O_2} and thus separately measure D_M and V_c.

Interpretation of Diffusing Capacity for CO

Table 5–1 shows that Elena's diffusing capacity for CO was greatly reduced from the predicted value of 25 to 11 ml · min^{-1} · mm Hg^{-1}. However, it should not be concluded that the whole of this reduction is caused by thickening of the blood-gas barrier and the reduction of capillary blood volume. It turns out that the measurement of diffusing capacity in a patient like this is affected by uneven ventilation and also by the distribution of diffusion properties, alveolar volume, and capillary blood. For this reason, the term *transfer factor* is sometimes used (particularly in Europe) to emphasize that the measurement does not solely reflect the diffusion properties of the lung.

Questions For each question, choose the one best answer.
(For answers, see p. 150.)

1. When a molecule of oxygen diffuses from the alveolar gas to the hemoglobin of a red blood cell through the thin side of the blood-gas barrier, all of the following are encountered EXCEPT:
   A. Layer of surfactant.
   B. Type I alveolar epithelial cell.
   C. Interstitium.
   D. Type I collagen fibers.
   E. Capillary endothelial cell.

2. A medical student develops a spontaneous pneumothorax because a bleb on the surface of one lung ruptures. All of the following are true of the affected side EXCEPT:
   A. Intrapleural pressure rises.
   B. Alveolar pressure rises.
   C. Chest wall moves out.
   D. Diaphragm moves down.
   E. Pulmonary blood flow decreases.

3. All of the following are true of the relaxation pressure-volume curve of the lung and chest wall EXCEPT:
   A. Relaxation pressure of the lung plus chest wall is zero at FRC.
   B. Relaxation pressure of the chest wall at FRC is less than atmospheric pressure.
   C. Relaxation pressure of the chest wall at TLC is above atmospheric pressure.
   D. Relaxation pressure of the lung at residual volume is zero.
   E. Relaxation pressure of the lung plus chest wall exceeds that of the lung alone at TLC.

4. In a patient with diffuse interstitial fibrosis of the lung, the maximal expiratory flow rate at a given lung volume may be higher than in a normal subject. Factors responsible for this include all of the following EXCEPT:
   A. Expiratory muscles have a large mechanical advantage.

   B. Airways have a large diameter.
   C. Dynamic compression of the airways is less likely than in a normal subject.
   D. Radial traction on the airways is increased.
   E. Airway resistance is decreased.

5. Carbon monoxide is used to measure the diffusing capacity of the lung because:
   A. It diffuses very slowly across the blood-gas barrier.
   B. It has a very low solubility in blood.
   C. The rate of combination of CO with hemoglobin is very rapid.
   D. Its partial pressure in blood at the end of the capillary is very low compared with that in alveolar gas.
   E. Its solubility in the blood-gas barrier is very high.

6. In a normal person, doubling the pulmonary diffusing capacity would be expected to:
   A. Increase the uptake of nitrous oxide given during anesthesia.
   B. Increase maximal oxygen uptake at extreme altitude.
   C. Increase resting arterial P_{O_2}.
   D. Decrease arterial P_{CO_2}.
   E. Increase resting oxygen uptake when the subject breathes 10% oxygen.

7. Factors that might lead to diffusion limitation of oxygen transfer across the blood-gas barrier include all of the following EXCEPT:
   A. Exercise.
   B. Fibrosis of the blood-gas barrier.
   C. Breathing a low oxygen mixture.
   D. High cardiac output.
   E. SCUBA diving.

8. **Which of the following statements about the diffusing capacity of the lung is FALSE?**

   A. It is best measured with carbon monoxide because this gas combines with hemoglobin 240 times faster than oxygen.

   B. Breathing oxygen reduces the measured diffusing capacity for carbon monoxide compared with air breathing.

   C. Diffusion limitation of oxygen transfer during exercise is more likely to occur at high altitude than sea level.

   D. It is decreased in pulmonary fibrosis.

   E. It is decreased by pneumonectomy (removal of one lung.)

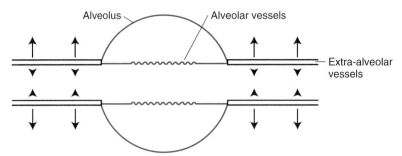

FIGURE 6–4. Alveolar and extra-alveolar vessels. The first vessels are mainly the capillaries and are exposed to alveolar pressure. The second vessels are pulled open by the radial traction of the sur- rounding lung parenchyma, and the effective pres- sure around them is therefore lower than alveolar pressure.

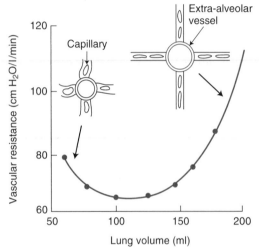

FIGURE 6–5. Effect of changes in lung volume on pulmonary vascular resistance when the transmu- ral pressure of the capillaries is held constant. At low lung volumes, resistance is high because the extra-alveolar vessels become narrow. At high lung volumes, the capillaries are stretched, and their caliber is reduced. (Data from an experimental animal.)

pressure, the vessels tend to be squashed, and their resistance rises. This usually occurs when a normal subject takes a deep inspiration, because the vascular pressures fall (the heart is sur- rounded by intrapleural pressure, which falls on inspiration). However, the pressures in the pulmonary circulation do not remain steady after such a maneuver. An additional factor that increases capillary resistance at large lung vol- umes is stretching and consequent thinning of the alveolar walls (Fig. 6–5). This has the effect of reducing the caliber of the capillaries and therefore increasing their resistance. Therefore,

even if the transmural pressure of the capillaries is not changed with large lung inflations, as was the case for the measurements shown in Figure 6–5, their vascular resistance increases.

Because of the role of smooth muscle in determining the caliber of the extra-alveolar vessels, drugs that cause contraction of this muscle increase pulmonary vascular resistance. These include serotonin, histamine, and norepi- nephrine. These drugs are particularly effective vasoconstrictors when the lung volume is low and the expanding forces on the vessels are weak. They are also very effective in the newborn lung because the pulmonary blood vessels in the fetus and newborn have large amounts of smooth muscle. Drugs that can relax smooth muscle in the pulmonary circulation include acetylcholine and isoproterenol.

Distribution of Pulmonary Blood Flow

So far we have been assuming that all parts of the pulmonary circulation behave identically. How- ever, considerable inequality of blood flow exists within the human lung. Indeed we have already referred to the preference of pulmonary emboli to lodge in the lower lobes.

The topographical inequality of blood flow in the lung can be measured using radioactive albumin aggregates (Fig. 6–1), or better, radio- active xenon. The gas is dissolved in saline and injected into a peripheral vein **(FIGURE 6–6)**. When it reaches the pulmonary capillaries, it is evolved into alveolar gas because of its low solubility, and the distribution of radioactivity can be measured by counters over the chest during breath-holding.

In the upright human lung, blood flow decreases almost linearly from bottom to top, reaching very low values at the apex (Fig. 6–6). This distribution is affected by change of posture and exercise. When the subject lies supine, the apical zone blood flow increases, but the basal zone flow remains virtually unchanged, with the result that the distribution from apex to base becomes almost uniform. However, in this posture, blood flow in the posterior (lower, or dependent) regions of the lung exceeds flow in the anterior parts. Measurements on subjects suspended upside down show that apical blood flow may exceed basal blood flow in this position. On mild exercise, both upper and lower zone blood flows increase and the regional differences become less.

The uneven distribution of blood flow can be explained by the hydrostatic pressure differences within the blood vessels. If we consider the pulmonary arterial system as a continuous column of blood, the difference in pressure between the top and bottom of the lung 30 cm high will be about 30 cm H_2O, or 23 mm Hg. This is a large pressure difference for such a low pressure system as the pulmonary circulation (*see* Fig. 1–10), and its effects on regional blood flow are shown in **FIGURE 6–7**.

There may be a region at the top of the lung (*zone 1*) where pulmonary arterial pressure falls below alveolar pressure (normally close to atmo-spheric pressure). If this occurs, the capillaries are squashed flat, and no flow is possible. This zone 1 does *not* occur under normal conditions, because the pulmonary arterial pressure is just sufficient to raise blood to the top of the lung, but may be present if the arterial pressure is reduced (following severe hemorrhage, for example), or if alveolar pressure is raised (during positive pressure ventilation). This ventilated but unperfused lung is useless for gas exchange and is called *alveolar dead space*.

Further down the lung (*zone 2*), pulmonary arterial pressure increases because of the hydro-static effect, and now exceeds alveolar pressure. However, venous pressure is still very low and is less than alveolar pressure, and this leads to remarkable pressure-flow characteristics. Under these conditions, blood flow is determined by the difference between the arterial and alveolar pressures (not the usual arterial-venous pressure difference). Indeed, venous pressure has no influence on flow unless it exceeds alveolar pressure.

This behavior can be modeled with a flexible rubber tube inside a glass chamber (**FIGURE 6–8**). When chamber pressure is greater than downstream pressure, the rubber tube collapses at its downstream end, and the pressure in the tube at this point limits flow. Of course, the pulmonary capillary bed is clearly very different from a rubber tube. Nevertheless, the overall

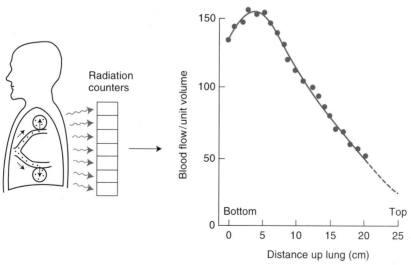

FIGURE 6–6. Measurement with radioactive xenon of the distribution of blood flow in the upright human lung. The dissolved xenon is evolved into alveolar gas from the pulmonary capillaries. The units of blood flow are such that if flow were uniform, all values would be 100. Note the small value at the apex.

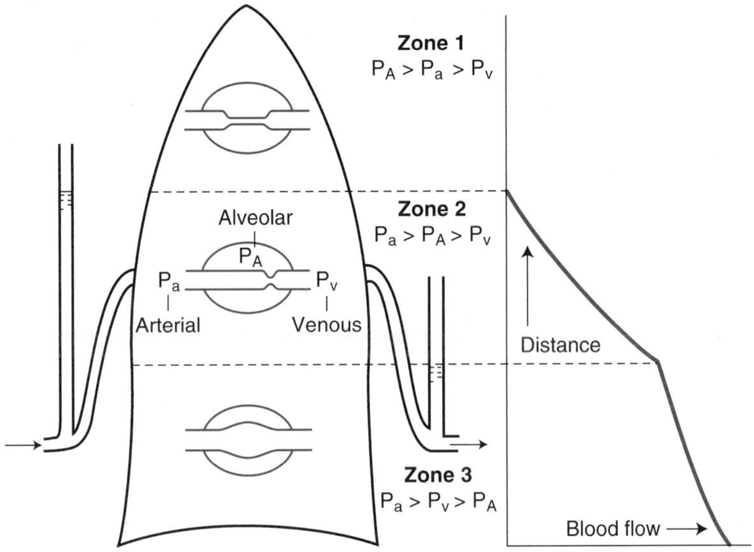

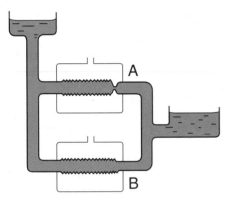

FIGURE 6–7. Explanation of the uneven distribution of blood flow in the lung based on the pressures affecting the capillaries. (See text for details.)

Zone 1
$P_A > P_a > P_v$

Zone 2
$P_a > P_A > P_v$

Alveolar
P_A

P_a P_v
Arterial   Venous

Distance

Zone 3
$P_a > P_v > P_A$

Blood flow →

FIGURE 6–8. Two Starling resistors, each consisting of a thin-walled rubber tube inside a container. When chamber pressure exceeds downstream pressure as in **A**, flow is independent of downstream pressure. However, when downstream pressure exceeds chamber pressure as in **B**, flow is determined by the upstream-downstream difference.

behavior is similar and this is often called the Starling resistor, sluice, or waterfall effect. Since arterial pressure is increasing down the zone but alveolar pressure is the same throughout the lung, the pressure difference responsible for flow increases. In addition, increasing recruitment of capillaries occurs down this zone.

Parenthetically, the same phenomenon occurs in the airways during a forced expiration. We saw in Figure 3–16 that once airway compression occurs, airflow is determined by the dif-

ference between alveolar pressure and the pressure outside the collapsed point. Recall that this is the reason why airflow rate is effort-independent during most of forced expiration.

In *zone 3*, venous pressure now exceeds alveolar pressure, and flow is determined in the usual way by the arterial-venous pressure difference. The increase in blood flow down this region of lung is apparently caused chiefly by distension of the capillaries. The pressure within them (lying between arterial and venous) increases down the zone, while the pressure outside them (alveolar) remains constant. Therefore, their transmural pressure rises and, indeed, measurements in animal preparations show that their mean width increases. Recruitment of previously closed vessels may also play some part in the increase in blood flow down this zone.

The scheme shown in Figure 6–7 summarizes the role played by the capillaries in determining the distribution of blood flow. At low lung volumes, the resistance of the extra-alveolar vessels becomes important, and a reduction of regional blood flow is seen, starting first at the base of the lung where the parenchyma is least well expanded (*see* Fig. 3–11). This region of reduced blood flow is sometimes called *zone 4*, and can be explained by the narrowing of the extra-alveolar vessels which occurs when the lung around them is poorly inflated (Fig. 6–5).

There are other factors that cause unevenness of blood flow in the lung. In some animals, some regions of the lung appear to have an intrinsically higher vascular resistance than others.

There is also evidence that blood flow decreases along the acinus, with peripheral parts less well supplied with blood. Some measurements suggest that the peripheral regions of the whole lung receive less blood flow than the central regions. Finally, the complex, partly random, arrangement of blood vessels and capillaries (*see* Fig. 1–11) causes some inequality of blood flow.

Active Control of the Circulation

We have seen that passive factors dominate the vascular resistance and the distribution of flow in the human pulmonary circulation under normal conditions. However, a remarkable active response occurs when the P_{O_2} of alveolar gas is reduced. This is known as *hypoxic pulmonary vasoconstriction* and was briefly referred to in Chapter 2. It consists of contraction of smooth muscle in the walls of the small arterioles in the hypoxic region. The precise mechanism of this response is still not known, but it occurs in excised isolated lung and so does not depend on central nervous connections. Excised segments of pulmonary artery can be shown to constrict if their environment is made hypoxic, so that it may be a local action of the hypoxia on the artery itself. One hypothesis is that cells in the perivascular tissue release some vasoconstrictor substance in response to hypoxia. Interestingly, it is the P_{O_2} of the alveolar gas, not the pulmonary arterial blood, that chiefly determines the response. This can be proved by perfusing a lung with blood of a high P_{O_2} while keeping the alveolar P_{O_2} low. Under these conditions the response occurs.

The vessel wall presumably becomes hypoxic through diffusion of oxygen over the very short distance from the wall to the surrounding alveoli. Recall that a small pulmonary artery is very closely surrounded by alveoli (compare the proximity of alveoli to the small pulmonary vein in Fig. 1–13). The stimulus-response curve of this hypoxic vasoconstriction is very nonlinear **(FIGURE 6–9)**. When the alveolar P_{O_2} is altered in the region above 100 mm Hg, little change in vascular resistance is seen. However, when the alveolar P_{O_2} is reduced below approximately 70 mm Hg, marked vasoconstriction may occur, and at a very low P_{O_2} the local blood flow may be almost abolished.

The mechanism of hypoxic pulmonary vasoconstriction remains obscure despite a great deal of research. Recent studies suggest that potassium ion channels in smooth muscle cells may be involved, leading to increased calcium ion concentrations within the cells.

Endothelium-derived vasoactive substances play a role. Nitric oxide (NO) has been shown to be an endothelium-derived relaxing factor for blood vessels. It is formed from L-arginine under the influence of the enzyme, nitric oxide synthase (NOS), and is a final common pathway for a variety of biological processes. NO activates soluble guanylate cyclase, which leads to smooth muscle relaxation through the synthesis of cyclic

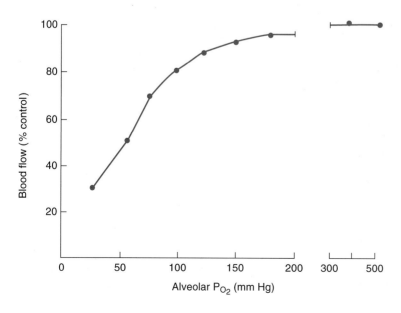

FIGURE 6–9. Effect of reducing the alveolar P_{O_2} on pulmonary blood flow. Note the very nonlinear response. (Data from an anesthetized cat.)

GMP. Inhibitors of NO synthesis augment hypoxic pulmonary vasoconstriction in animal preparations, and inhaled NO reduces hypoxic pulmonary vasoconstriction in humans. The required inhaled concentration of NO is extremely low (about 10 to 20 ppm), and the gas is very toxic at high concentrations.

Pulmonary vascular endothelial cells also release potent vasoconstrictor peptides known as endothelins. Their role in normal physiology and disease is the subject of intense study.

Hypoxic vasoconstriction has the effect of directing blood flow away from hypoxic regions of lung. These regions may result from local airway obstruction (see Figs. 3–18 and 4–13), and by diverting blood flow the deleterious effects on gas exchange are reduced. We saw in Chapter 2 that at high altitude, generalized pulmonary vasoconstriction may occur, leading to a large rise in pulmonary arterial pressure. However, probably the most important situation where this mechanism operates is at birth. During fetal life, the pulmonary vascular resistance is very high, partly because of hypoxic vasoconstriction, and only some 15% of the cardiac output goes through the lungs. The rest bypasses the lungs through the patent ductus arteriosus. When the first breath oxygenates the alveoli, the vascular resistance falls dramatically because of relaxation of vascular smooth muscle, and the pulmonary blood flow increases enormously.

Other active responses of the pulmonary circulation have been described. A low blood pH causes vasoconstriction, especially when alveolar hypoxia is present. There is also evidence that the autonomic nervous system exerts a weak control, an increase in sympathetic outflow causing stiffening of the walls of the pulmonary arteries and vasoconstriction.

Metabolic Functions of the Pulmonary Circulation

TABLE 6–1 shows that a number of vasoactive substances are metabolized by the lung. Since the lung is the only organ except the heart that receives the whole circulation, it is uniquely suited to modifying blood-borne substances. A substantial fraction of all the vascular endothelial cells in the body are located in the lung.

The only known example of biological activation by passage through the pulmonary circulation is the conversion of the relatively inactive polypeptide, angiotensin I, to the potent vaso-

TABLE 6–1
Fate of Substances in the Pulmonary Circulation

Substance	Fate
Peptides	
Angiotensin I	Converted to angiotensin II by ACE
Angiotensin II	Unaffected
Vasopressin	Unaffected
Bradykinin	Up to 80% inactivated
Amines	
Serotonin	Almost completely removed
Norepinephrine	Up to 30% removed
Histamine	Not affected
Dopamine	Not affected
Arachidonic Acid Metabolites	
Prostaglandin E_2 and $F_{2\alpha}$	Almost completely removed
Prostaglandin A_2	Not affected
Prostacyclin (PGI_2)	Not affected
Leukotrienes	Almost completely removed

constrictor, angiotensin II. The latter, which is up to 50 times more active than its precursor, is unaffected by passage through the lung. The conversion of angiotensin I is catalyzed by an enzyme, angiotensin-converting enzyme (ACE), which is located in small pits on the surface of the capillary endothelial cells.

Many vasoactive substances are completely or partially inactivated during passage through the lung. Bradykinin is largely inactivated (up to 80%), and the enzyme responsible is ACE. The lung is the major site of inactivation of serotonin (5-hydroxytryptamine), but this is not by enzymatic degradation, but by an uptake and storage process. Some of the serotonin may be transferred to platelets in the lung, or stored in some other way and released during anaphylaxis. The prostaglandins E_1, E_2, and $F_{2\alpha}$ are also inactivated in the lung which is a rich source of the responsible enzymes. Norepinephrine is also taken up by the lung to some extent (up to 30%). Histamine appears not to be affected by the intact lung but is readily inactivated by slices.

Some vasoactive materials pass through the lung without significant gain or loss of activity. These include epinephrine, prostaglandins A_1 and A_2, angiotensin II, and vasopressin (ADH).

Several vasoactive and bronchoactive substances are metabolized in the lung and may be released into the circulation under certain conditions. Important among these are the arachidonic acid metabolites **(FIGURE 6–10)**. Arachidonic acid is formed through the action of the enzyme phospholipase A_2 on phospholipid bound to cell membranes. There are two major synthetic pathways, the initial reactions being catalyzed by the enzymes lipoxygenase and cyclooxygenase, respectively. The first produces the leukotrienes which include the mediator originally described as slow-reacting substance of anaphylaxis (SRS-A). These compounds cause airway constriction and may have an important role in asthma, as described in Chapter 4. Other leukotrienes are involved in inflammatory responses.

The prostaglandins are potent vasoconstrictors or vasodilators. PGE_2 plays an important role in the perinatal period, because it helps to relax the patent ductus arteriosus. Prostaglandins also affect platelet aggregation and are active in other systems, such as the kallikrein-kinin clotting cascade. They also may have a role in the bronchoconstriction of asthma.

Surface Tension and Surfactant

We have seen that Fiona's pulmonary embolism resolved well following treatment with anticoagulants. The emboli are removed by circulating fibrinolytic enzymes, and the appearance of the pulmonary blood vessels may be completely normal a few weeks after the embolic events. In her case, there were no complications in the embolized regions, and the chest radiograph remained essentially normal, except for a slight reduction of vascular markings in the embolized area.

In some patients, a pulmonary embolus is complicated by alveolar hemorrhage and atelec-tasis of the embolized region. Rarely, pulmonary infarction occurs with death of the embolized tissue. There is alveolar filling with extravasated red cells and inflammatory cells, and an opacity is seen on the radiograph. Rarely the infarct may become infected, leading to an abscess. The infrequency of these complications can be explained, in part, by the fact that most emboli do not obstruct the vessel completely. In addition, bronchial artery anastomoses and the airways supply oxygen to the lung parenchyma.

In experimental animals, ligation of a lobar pulmonary artery can lead to atelectasis with extravasation of red cells in the affected lobe. It has been shown that these changes are caused by the loss of surfactant. Surfactant metabolism is a vital function of the pulmonary circulation, and this is a convenient place to discuss surfactant and surface tension in the lung. These topics were referred to in Chapter 3 when the pressure-volume behavior of the lung was discussed (*see* Fig. 3–9). It was pointed out there that the elastic recoil of the lung depends on two basic factors: (1) the elastin and collagen fibers within the lung substance, and (2) the surface tension of the alveolar lining layer.

Surface tension is a difficult concept for some people and so a brief introduction may be helpful. Surface tension is defined as the force (in dynes, for example) acting across an imaginary line 1 cm long in the surface of a liquid **(FIGURE 6–11A)**. It arises because the attractive forces between adjacent molecules of the liquid are much stronger than those between molecules of the liquid and overlying gas, with the result that the liquid surface area becomes as small as possible. In fact we can think of the surface tension as similar to the tension in a thin sheet of rubber stretched across the trough shown in Figure 6–11A. Now suppose we make a 1-cm long incision in the rubber sheet. This will cause it to gape. If we then take sutures

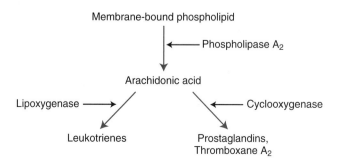

FIGURE 6–10. Two pathways of arachidonic acid metabolism. The leukotrienes are generated by the lipoxygenase pathway, while the prostaglandins and thromboxane A_2 come from the cyclooxygenase pathway.

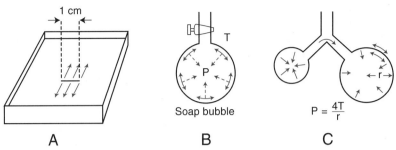

FIGURE 6–11. A. Surface tension is the force (in dynes, for example) acting across an imaginary line 1 cm long in a liquid surface. **B.** Surface forces in a soap bubble tend to reduce the area of the surface and generate a pressure within the bubble. **C.** Because the smaller bubble generates a larger pressure, it blows up the larger bubble.

and close the gaping hole, the total force acting on the sutures is analogous to the surface tension.

Some of the properties of surface tension can be seen if we blow a soap bubble on the end of a tube (Fig. 6–11B). The surfaces of the bubble contract as much as they can, forming a sphere (smallest surface area for a given volume), and generating a pressure (P) that can be predicted from Laplace's law:

$$P = \frac{4 \cdot T}{r}$$

where T is the surface tension and r is the radius. When only one surface is involved, for example, in a liquid-lined spherical alveolus, the numerator is 2 rather than 4.

The first evidence that surface tension contributes to the pressure-volume behavior of lung was obtained by von Neergaard when he showed that lungs inflated with saline have a much larger compliance (are easier to distend) than air-filled lungs **(FIGURE 6–12)**. Since the saline abolished the surface tension forces but presumably did not affect the tissue forces of the lung, this observation meant that surface tension contributed part of the static recoil force of the lung. Some time later, workers studying edema foam coming from the lungs of animals exposed to noxious gases noted that the tiny air bubbles of the foam were extremely stable. They recognized that this indicated a very low surface tension, an observation which led to the remarkable discovery of *pulmonary surfactant*.

It is now known that type II alveolar epithelial cells (*see* Fig. 5–3) secrete a material that profoundly lowers the surface tension of the alveolar lining fluid. Recall that the type II cells contain prominent lamellated bodies (*see* Fig. 5–3). These contain phospholipid, which is formed in the endoplasmic reticulum, passed through the Golgi apparatus, and eventually extruded into the alveolar space to form surfactant. The exact nature of surfactant is not known, but dipalmitoyl phosphatidylcholine (DPPC) is an important constituent. Some of the surfactant can be washed out of lungs by rinsing them with saline.

The phospholipid DPPC is synthesized in the lung from fatty acids that are either extracted from the blood or are themselves synthesized in the lung. Synthesis is fast, and there is a rapid turnover of surfactant. If the blood flow to a region of lung is abolished as a result of an embolus, the surfactant is depleted. Surfactant is formed relatively late in fetal life, and babies born without adequate amounts develop infant respiratory distress syndrome and may die.

The effects of surfactant on surface tension can be studied with a surface balance **(FIGURE 6–13)**. This consists of a trough containing saline on which a small amount of test material is placed. The area of the surface is then alternately expanded and compressed by a movable barrier while the surface tension is measured from the force exerted on a platinum strip dipped into the surface. Pure saline gives a surface tension of about 70 dynes $\cdot$ cm^{-1}, irrespective of the area of its surface. Adding detergent to the saline reduces the surface tension, but again this is independent of area. When lung washings are placed on saline, the curve shown in Figure 6–13B is obtained. The surface tension changes greatly with the surface area, and there is hysteresis (compare Figs. 3–9 and 6–12). In addition, the surface tension falls to extremely low values when the area is small.

How does surfactant reduce the surface tension so much? A simple explanation is that the molecules of DPPC are hydrophobic at one end and hydrophilic at the other, and they therefore align themselves in the surface. When this occurs, their intermolecular repulsive forces oppose the normal attracting forces between surface molecules that are responsible for surface tension. The reduction in surface tension is greatest when the film is compressed because the molecules of DPPC are then crowded closer together and repel each other more.

What are the physiological advantages of surfactant? First, a low surface tension in the alveoli increases the compliance of the lung and reduces the work of expanding it with each breath. Second, stability of the alveoli is promoted. The 300 million alveoli appear to be inherently unstable because areas of atelectasis often form in the presence of disease. This is a complex subject, but one way of looking at the lung is to regard it as a collection of millions of tiny bubbles (although this is an oversimplification). In such an arrangement, there is a tendency for small bubbles to collapse and blow up large ones. Figure 6–11C shows that the pressure generated by the surface forces in a bubble is inversely proportional to its radius, with the result that if the surface tensions are the same, the pressure inside a small bubble exceeds that in a large bubble. However, Figure 6–13 shows that when lung washings are present, a

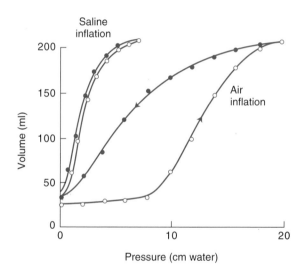

FIGURE 6–12. Comparison of pressure-volume curves of air-filled and saline-filled lungs. *Open circles*, inflation; *closed circles*, deflation. The saline-filled lung has a higher compliance and much less hysteresis than the air-filled lung. (Data from an animal preparation.)

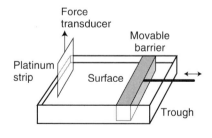

A

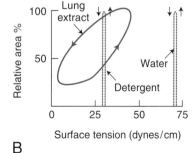

B

FIGURE 6–13. A. Surface balance. The area of the surface is altered by moving the barrier, and the surface tension is measured from the force exerted on a platinum strip dipped into the surface. **B.** Plots of surface tension and area obtained with a surface balance. Note that lung washings show a change in the surface tension with area and that the minimum tension is very small.

small surface area is associated with a small surface tension. Thus, the tendency for small alveoli to empty into large alveoli is apparently reduced.

A third role of surfactant is to help to keep the alveoli dry. This is a difficult concept, but just as the surface tension forces tend to collapse alveoli, they also tend to suck fluid out of the capillaries. In effect, the surface tension of the curved alveolar surface reduces the hydrostatic pressure in the tissue outside the capillaries. By reducing these surface forces, surfactant inhibits the transudation of fluid.

What are the consequences of absence of surfactant? On the basis of its functions discussed above, we would expect these to be stiff lungs (low compliance), areas of atelectasis, and alveoli filled with transudate. Indeed, these are the pathophysiological features of infant respiratory distress syndrome **(FIGURE 6–14)**, and this disease is caused by an absence of this crucial material. The same changes occur in the lobe of

an experimental animal lung after ligation of the lobar pulmonary artery.

Other Pathophysiological Changes in Pulmonary Embolism

Gas Exchange

Patients with pulmonary embolism typically have a reduced arterial P_{O_2} but a normal P_{CO_2}. This was the case with Fiona, whose P_{O_2} was 78 mm Hg (normal >90), P_{CO_2} was 38 mm Hg, and pH was 7.41. Measurements by the multiple inert gas elimination technique (*see* Figs. 3–22 and 3–23) show that the hypoxemia can often be explained by ventilation-perfusion inequality, although some patients, particularly those with very large emboli, have large shunts. One mechanism for the shunt is blood flow through atelectatic areas, as referred to above. However, some patients with massive pulmonary embolism also develop some alveolar edema. The

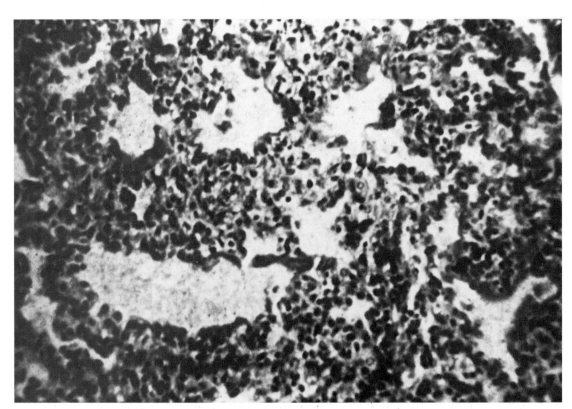

FIGURE 6–14. Microscopic section of lung from a premature baby with infant respiratory distress syndrome. There are areas of atelectasis and hemorrhagic edema. The lung was also difficult to inflate. These are the consequences of the absence of surfactant.

probable explanation is that the high pulmonary artery pressure raises the pressure in capillaries in nonembolized areas of lung, and these capillaries leak fluid into the alveolar spaces. The pathogenesis of pulmonary edema is discussed in detail in Chapter 7. The arterial P_{CO_2} after pulmonary embolism is maintained at the normal level by an increase in ventilation to the alveoli. This increase may be substantial because of the large physiological dead space, and therefore wasted ventilation, caused by the embolized area.

Lung Mechanics

If a pulmonary artery is occluded by a catheter in experimental animals, the ventilation to that area of lung is often reduced. The mechanism is a direct effect of the reduced arterial P_{CO_2} on the smooth muscle of the local small airways, causing bronchoconstriction. It can be reversed by adding CO_2 to the inspired gas. Although this airway response to vascular obstruction is much weaker than the corresponding vascular response to airway obstruction (hypoxic pulmonary vasoconstriction) it serves a similar homeostatic role. The reduction in airflow to the unperfused lung reduces the amount of wasted ventilation and thus the physiological dead space. This reduction of ventilation is apparently absent or short-lived after pulmonary thromboembolism in humans because most measurements of the distribution of ventilation with radioactive xenon made some hours after the episode show no ventilation defect in the embolized area. This was the case in Fiona, as shown in Figure 6–1.

Cardiovascular Changes

Massive emboli may produce sudden hemodynamic collapse with central chest pain, rapid weak pulse, hypotension, and neck vein engorgement. As discussed earlier, repeated small emboli may result in severe pulmonary hypertension.

Questions

For each question, choose the one best answer.
(For answers, see p. 150.)

1. Clinical features of pulmonary embolism may typically include all of the following EXCEPT:
   A. Hemoptysis
   B. Rigor (shivering attack)
   C. Pleuritic pain
   D. Dyspnea
   E. Loud pulmonary second sound

2. Factors that increase the likelihood of formation of peripheral venous thrombi include all of the following EXCEPT:
   A. Polycythemia
   B. Use of oral contraceptives
   C. Medication with aspirin
   D. Immobilization of a limb
   E. Dehydration

3. Pulmonary vascular resistance is reduced by:
   A. Acute narrowing of the mitral valve
   B. Removal of one lung
   C. Positive pressure mechanical ventilation
   D. Breathing a 10% oxygen mixture
   E. Exhaling from FRC to residual volume.

4. In the normal human, systemic vascular resistance exceeds pulmonary vascular resistance how many fold?
   A. 2
   B. 4
   C. 6
   D. 8
   E. 10

5. In zone 2 of the lung:
   A. The capillaries are closed.
   B. The pressure difference responsible for blood flow increases down the lung.
   C. Distension of capillaries is the main factor responsible for the increase in blood flow down the lung.
   D. Blood flow is determined by the arterial-venous pressure difference.
   E. Pulmonary venous pressure exceeds alveolar pressure.

6. A patient's lung is inflated by positive pressure using a mechanical ventilator. All the following are true EXCEPT:
   A. Pulmonary vascular resistance increases.
   B. The caliber of the extra-alveolar vessels increases.
   C. Venous return to the thorax is impeded.
   D. The caliber of the pulmonary capillaries is reduced.
   E. The likelihood of zone 1 conditions occurring is reduced.

7. An isolated ventilated lung is perfused by gravity from a reservoir at a fixed height. The reservoir contains normal venous blood, and the ventilation and blood flow are initially set to give normal arterial blood gas values. All of the following would be expected EXCEPT:
   A. If the ventilation is halved, the blood flow decreases.
   B. If the ventilation is halved, the arterial pH falls.
   C. If the height of the reservoir is halved, blood flow is halved.
   D. If the height of the reservoir is increased, pulmonary vascular resistance decreases.
   E. Changing the ventilating gas from air to 10% oxygen decreases blood flow.

8. The following statements about hypoxic pulmonary vasoconstriction are true EXCEPT:
   A. Its mechanism involves K^+ channels in vascular smooth muscle.
   B. It depends more on the P_{O_2} of mixed venous blood than alveolar gas.
   C. It is important in the transition from placental to air respiration.
   D. It partly diverts blood flow from poorly ventilated regions of diseased lungs.
   E. It is important in the development of high-altitude pulmonary edema.

9. **Which of the following statements about pulmonary capillaries is FALSE?**
   A. The endothelial cells contain angiotensin-converting enzyme.
   B. Average diffusing distance from alveolar epithelial cells to red blood cell in the lung is less than from capillary endothelial cell to mitochondria in leg muscle.
   C. Diameter of capillaries increases when their transmural pressure increases.
   D. When blood passes through them, bradykinin in the blood is largely inactivated.
   E. Pulmonary venous pressure may exceed capillary pressure in mid-lung during vigorous exercise.

10. **Metabolic functions of the pulmonary circulation include all of the following EXCEPT:**
    A. Removal of prostaglandin E_2
    B. Partial removal of norepinephrine
    C. Inactivation of vasopressin
    D. Partial inactivation of bradykinin
    E. Conversion of angiotensin I to angiotensin II

11. **The following statements about nitric oxide in the lung are true EXCEPT:**
    A. It causes relaxation of smooth muscle by reducing the concentration of cyclic GMP.
    B. It is formed from L-arginine.
    C. Enzymatic control of its synthesis is by nitric oxide synthase.
    D. Inhaled NO reduces hypoxic pulmonary vasoconstriction.
    E. Inhaled NO is biologically active at concentrations of less than 50 parts per million.

12. **The following statements about pulmonary surfactant are true EXCEPT:**
    A. It contains dipalmitoyl phosphatidyl choline.
    B. It is rapidly turned over in the lung.
    C. It reduces the hydrostatic pressure outside the pulmonary capillaries.
    D. It is stored in alveolar type II epithelial cells as laminated bodies.
    E. It results in air-filled lung having a lower compliance than saline-filled lung.

13. **Some newborn infants lack pulmonary surfactant. The consequences include all of the following EXCEPT:**
    A. Edema fluid in the alveoli
    B. Areas of atelectasis
    C. The lungs are difficult to inflate
    D. Atrophy of the respiratory muscles
    E. Severe arterial hypoxemia

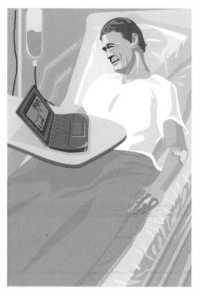

Chapter 7

Pulmonary Edema

☐ George is a 55-year-old stockbroker who developed a myocardial infarction which caused left heart failure and pulmonary edema. We discuss the physiology of fluid movement across the walls of pulmonary capillaries and the pathophysiology of the various types of pulmonary edema. George has arterial hypoxemia as a result of blood flow through nonventilated areas of lung, and the physiology of shunt is also discussed.

☐ CLINICAL FINDINGS

History

George is a 55-year-old stockbroker who was well until 3 years when he began to have central chest discomfort during physical exertion such as playing golf. He did not seek medical advice. On the morning of hospital admission he had an attack of severe central chest pain which he described as crushing and which radiated into his left shoulder. Shortly after this he became very short of breath and coughed up a small amount of frothy fluid. He was admitted to the hospital as an emergency. There was no history of shortness of breath or ankle swelling. He smoked a pack of cigarettes a day for the past 35 years. His family history is significant, in that his father died of a heart attack at the age of 60 and George's 50-year-old brother has had heart problems. George's job as a stockbroker causes him much anxiety at times, and he worries a lot.

Physical Examination

In the emergency department the patient appeared anxious and was short of breath. He coughed up small amounts of pink frothy fluid. His temperature was 38°C, blood pressure 110/65 mm Hg, pulse 100 beats · min^{-1}. There

was facial pallor and some sweating, but no neck vein engorgement. The apex beat of the heart was in the 5th intercostal space in the midclavicular line. The heart sounds were soft with a gallop rhythm (that is, three rather than two heart sounds could be heard). On auscultation of the chest, rales (crackles) could be heard at the bases of both lungs posteriorly. The liver was not palpable, and there was no ankle or sacral edema.

Investigations

An electrocardiogram (ECG) showed the pattern of a recent left anterior wall infarct with Q waves and depressed ST segments. A chest radiograph (FIGURE 7–1) showed blotchy bilateral opacities typical of pulmonary edema. Arterial blood gases showed a P_{O_2} of 59 mm Hg, P_{CO_2} of 35 mm Hg, and pH of 7.35.

Treatment and Progress

The patient was treated with bed rest, morphine, diuretics, and oxygen by nasal cannulas. His condition improved and the signs of pulmonary edema disappeared over 2 days. He had a coronary angiogram, which showed severe obstruction of the left anterior descending coronary artery. An operation for a coronary artery

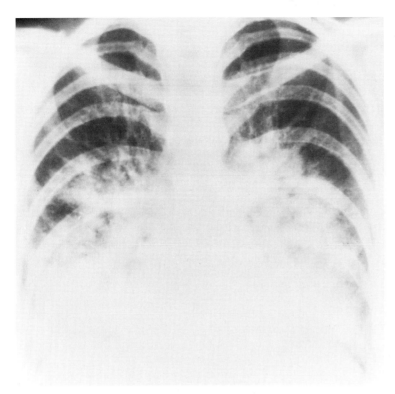

FIGURE 7–1. Chest radiograph of a patient with severe alveolar edema. Note the blotchy shadowing in both lungs.

bypass graft was performed and the patient made an uneventful recovery. The patient was advised to stop smoking.

Diagnosis

Pulmonary edema caused by left ventricular failure following a myocardial infarction.

☐ PHYSIOLOGY AND PATHOPHYSIOLOGY

Clinical Findings

George's clinical course is common enough, and it introduces us to many aspects of the pathophysiology of left ventricular failure and pulmonary edema. Starting with the clinical history, it is probable in retrospect that George had coronary artery disease for several years and that the pain he experienced during exertion was angina. The attack on the day of hospital admission was a myocardial infarction as a result of occlusion of part of his left anterior descending coronary artery. This resulted in anginal pain, ischemia of part of the left ventricular wall, failure of that portion of the myocardium to contract, and consequent pump failure of the left heart. The result was that blood dammed up behind the failing ventricle, causing an increase in left atrial and pulmonary venous pressures. These in turn raised pulmonary capillary pressure, and the result was alveolar pulmonary edema. The gallop rhythm heard on auscultation of the heart is common in myocardial infarction, and the rales heard over the lung bases were caused by fluid in the airways. The fact that he coughed up some blood-tinged frothy fluid meant that he had a severe attack of edema, but fortunately this responded to treatment.

We saw in Figure 1–10 that the normal mean pressure in the left atrium is about 5 mm Hg. When the left ventricle fails, this pressure rises as does the pressure in the pulmonary veins and the capillaries. As a result, the capillaries distend and some additional capillaries open up (*see* Fig. 6–3), and pulmonary artery pressure rises though not as much as pulmonary venous pressure because vascular resistance is decreased. However, the net result is that the hydrostatic pressure in the capillaries increases and fluid moves out of them.

Pulmonary Edema

A review of Figure 1–7 reminds us that the pulmonary capillaries are lined by endothelial cells and surrounded by an interstitial space. As shown in the figure, the interstitium is often narrow on one side of the capillary, where it is formed by the fusion of the basement membranes of the capillary endothelial and alveolar epithelial cells, while on the other side it is wider and contains some type I collagen fibers and a few cells such as fibroblasts. This wider side is particularly important for fluid exchange. Between the interstitium and the alveolar space is the alveolar epithelium composed predominantly of type I cells. There is also a thin layer of surfactant which is not shown in Figure 1–7 because it was removed by the fixation process.

The capillary endothelium is highly permeable to water and to many solutes, including small molecules and ions. Proteins have a restricted movement across the endothelium. By contrast, the alveolar epithelium is much less permeable, and even small ions are largely prevented from crossing by passive diffusion. In addition, the epithelium actively pumps water from the alveolar to the interstitial space using a sodium, potassium, ATPase pump.

Hydrostatic forces tend to move fluid out of the capillary into the interstitial space, while osmotic forces tend to keep it in. The movement of fluid across the endothelium is governed by the Starling equation:

$$\dot{Q} = K[(P_c - P_i) - \sigma(\pi_c - \pi_i)]$$

where $\dot{Q}$ is the net flow out of the capillary, K is the filtration coefficient, P_c and P_i are the hydrostatic pressures in the capillary and interstitial space respectively, π_c and π_i are the corresponding colloid osmotic pressures, and σ is the reflection coefficient. This last variable indicates the effectiveness of the membrane in preventing (reflecting) the passage of protein compared with water across the endothelium, and the coefficient is reduced in diseases that damage the endothelial cells and increase their permeability.

Although this equation is valuable conceptually, its practical use is limited. Of the four pressures, only one, the colloid osmotic pressure within the capillary, is known with any certainty. Its value is approximately 28 mm Hg. The capillary hydrostatic pressure is probably halfway between arterial and venous pressures (*see* Fig. 1–10), but varies markedly from top to bottom of the upright lung (*see* Fig. 6–7). The colloid osmotic pressure of the interstitial fluid is not known, but is approximately 20 mm Hg in lung lymph. However, there is some question about whether this lymph has the same protein concentration as the interstitial fluid around the capillaries. The interstitial hydrostatic pressure is unknown but is thought to be substantially below atmospheric pressure. The value of sigma (σ) in the pulmonary capillaries is approximately 0.7. It is probable that the net pressure from the Starling equilibrium is outward, causing a lymph flow of perhaps 20 ml · hr^{-1}.

The fluid that leaves the capillaries moves within the interstitial space of the alveolar wall and tracks to the perivascular and peribronchial interstitium (**FIGURE 7–2**). This tissue normally forms a thin sheath around the pulmonary arteries, veins, and bronchi and contains the lymphatics (*see* Fig. 1–13). The alveoli themselves are devoid of lymphatics, but once the fluid reaches the perivascular and peribronchial interstitium, some of it is carried in the lymphatics while some moves through the loose interstitial tissue. The lymphatics actively pump the lymph toward the bronchial and hilar lymph nodes.

If excessive amounts of fluid leak from the capillaries, two factors tend to limit this flow. The first is a fall in the colloid osmotic pressure of the interstitial fluid as the protein is diluted because of the faster filtration of water compared with protein. However, this factor does not operate if the permeability of the capillary is greatly increased. The second is the rise in hydrostatic pressure in the interstitial space, which reduces the net filtration pressure. Both factors act in a direction to reduce fluid movement out of the capillaries.

Two stages in the formation of pulmonary edema are recognized (Fig. 7–2). The first is interstitial edema, which is characterized by engorgement of the perivascular and peribronchial interstitial tissue (cuffing), as shown in **FIGURE 7–3**. Dilated lymphatics can be seen, and lymph flow increases. In addition, some widening of the interstitium of the alveolar wall on the thick side occurs. Pulmonary function is little affected at this stage, and the condition is difficult to recognize although some changes in the chest radiograph may be seen (see below).

The second stage is alveolar edema. Here, fluid moves across the alveoli which are filled one by one (**FIGURE 7-4**). As a result of surface tension forces, the edematous alveoli shrink in size. Ventilation is prevented, and to the extent that the alveoli remain perfused, shunting

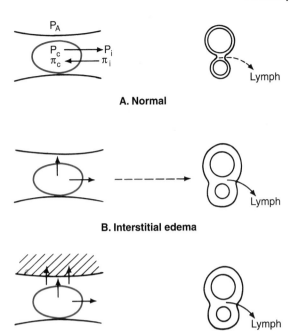

A. Normal

B. Interstitial edema

C. Alveolar edema

FIGURE 7-2. Stages of pulmonary edema. **A.** There is normally a small lymph flow from the lung. **B.** In interstitial edema there is an increased lymph flow with engorgement of the perivascular and peribronchial spaces and some widening of the interstitium of the alveolar wall. **C.** Some fluid crosses the blood-gas barrier producing alveolar edema.

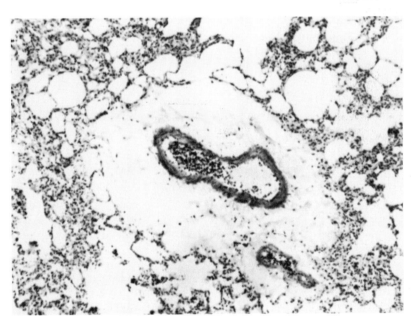

FIGURE 7-3. Example of engorgement of the perivascular space of a small pulmonary blood vessel by interstitial edema. Some alveolar edema is also present.

of blood occurs and arterial hypoxemia is inevitable (see below). The edema fluid may move into the small and large airways and be coughed up as voluminous frothy sputum. As we saw earlier, George coughed up some red-tinged frothy fluid. The red staining comes from the presence of red blood cells. What prompts the transition from interstitial to alveolar edema is not fully understood, but it may be that the lymphatics become overloaded and the pres-

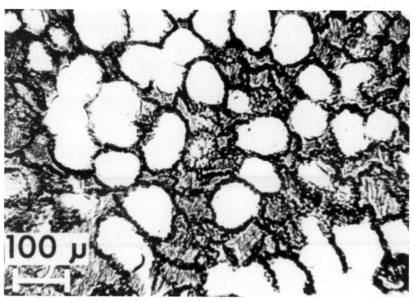

FIGURE 7–4. Histological appearance of alveolar edema. Some alveoli are completely filled, while others are spared. The edematous alveoli tend to be smaller.

sure in the interstitial space increases so much that fluid spills over into the alveoli. Probably the alveolar epithelium is damaged, and its permeability is increased. This would explain the presence of protein and red cells in the alveolar fluid. As indicated above, the alveolar epithelium is normally very effective in preventing the passage of protein, cells, and fluid across it.

Causes of Pulmonary Edema

These are best discussed under the following six headings (as also shown in **TABLE 7–1.**

Increased Capillary Hydrostatic Pressure

This is the most common cause of pulmonary edema and was also the cause in George's case. Here the precipitating event was left ventricular failure caused by an acute myocardial infarction, but hypertensive left ventricular failure and mitral valve disease are other causes. In all these conditions, left atrial pressure rises resulting in an increase in pulmonary venous and capillary pressures. This can be recognized at cardiac catheterization by measuring the "wedge" or

TABLE 7–1
Causes of Pulmonary Edema

Mechanism	Precipitating Event
Increased capillary hydrostatic pressure	Myocardial infarction, mitral stenosis, fluid overload, pulmonary veno-occlusive disease
Increased capillary permeability	Inhaled or circulating toxins, sepsis, radiation oxygen toxicity, ARDS
Reduced lymph drainage	Increased central venous pressure, lymphangitis carcinomatosa
?Decreased interstitial pressure	Rapid removal of pleural effusion or pneumothorax, hyperinflation
Decreased colloid osmotic pressure	Overtransfusion hypoalbuminemia, renal disease
Uncertain etiology	High altitude, neurogenic, overinflation, heroin

occlusion pressure (the pressure in a catheter that has been wedged in and, therefore, has blocked a small pulmonary artery). This pressure is approximately equal to pulmonary venous pressure.

Whether pulmonary edema occurs in these conditions depends partly on the rate of rise of the pressure. For example, in patients with mitral stenosis in whom the venous pressure gradually rises over a period of years, remarkably high values can occur without clinical evidence of edema. This is partly because the caliber, or number, of the lymphatics increase to accommodate the higher lymph flow. However, these patients often have marked interstitial edema. By contrast, a patient like George who had an acute myocardial infarction may develop alveolar edema with a smaller but more sudden rise in capillary pressure.

Noncardiogenic causes also occur. For example, edema may be precipitated by excess intravenous infusions of saline, plasma, or blood, leading to a rise in pulmonary capillary pressure. Diseases of the pulmonary veins, such as pulmonary veno-occlusive disease which results in blocked veins, may also result in edema.

An important mechanism of the edema in all these conditions is the increase in hydrostatic pressure in the capillaries because this disturbs the Starling equilibrium. However, recent work shows that when the capillary pressure is raised to unphysiologically high levels, ultrastructural changes occur in the capillary walls, including disruption of the capillary endothelium, alveolar epithelium, or sometimes all layers of the wall. The result is an increase in capillary permeability, with the movement of fluid, protein, and cells into the alveolar spaces. This condition is known as capillary stress failure.

One consequence of these changes in structure of the capillary wall is that for relatively small increases in pressure, the edema fluid has a low protein concentration because the permeability characteristics of the capillary wall are largely preserved (low-permeability edema). However, with large increases of capillary pressure, the protein concentration of the edema fluid is high (high-permeability edema) because the capillary walls are damaged.

Increased Capillary Permeability

Apart from the situation referred to above, an increased capillary permeability also occurs in a variety of other conditions. Inhaled toxins, such as chlorine, sulfur dioxide, or nitrogen oxides, can damage the pulmonary capillaries. Circulating toxins, such as alloxan or endotoxin, can cause pulmonary edema in the same way. Therapeutic radiation to the lung may cause edema and, ultimately, interstitial fibrosis. Oxygen poisoning produces a similar picture. Increased permeability is frequently seen in adult respiratory distress syndrome (ARDS; *see* Chapter 9). The edema fluid typically has a high protein concentration and contains many blood cells.

Reduced Lymph Drainage

This can be an exaggerating factor if another cause is present. Increased central venous pressure may occur in ARDS, heart failure, and overtransfusion and can interfere with the normal drainage of the thoracic duct. Obstruction of lymphatics, as in lymphangitis carcinomatosa, is another exaggerating cause.

Decreased Interstitial Pressure

This might be expected to promote edema from the Starling equation, although whether this occurs in practice is uncertain. However, unilateral pulmonary edema is sometimes seen in patients who have a large unilateral pleural effusion or pneumothorax, and then the lung is rapidly expanded. In this case the edema may be partly related to the large mechanical forces acting on the interstitial space as the lung is inflated. However, the edema fluid is of the high-permeability type, and it is probable that the high mechanical stresses in the alveolar walls cause ultrastructural changes in the capillary walls (stress failure).

Decreased Colloid Osmotic Pressure

This is rarely responsible for pulmonary edema on its own, but it can exaggerate the edema that occurs when some other precipitating factor is present. Overtransfusion with saline is an important example. This may occur in the management of ARDS. Another example is the hypoproteinemia of the nephrotic syndrome.

Uncertain Etiology

High-altitude pulmonary edema occasionally affects climbers and skiers and was referred to in Chapter 2. The pulmonary wedge pressure is normal, so a raised pulmonary venous pressure can be ruled out. However, the pulmonary artery pressure is high because of hypoxic pulmonary vasoconstriction (*see* Fig. 6–9). A current hypothesis is that the arteriolar constriction is uneven and that regions of the capillary bed which are therefore not protected from the high pressure develop the ultrastructural changes of stress failure. This hypothesis would explain the high protein concentration in the alveolar fluid. Treatment is by descent to a lower altitude. Oxygen should be given if available.

Neurogenic pulmonary edema is seen after injuries to the brain (for example, head trauma). Again the mechanism is probably stress failure of pulmonary capillaries because it is known that there is a large rise in capillary pressure associated with heightened activity of the sympathetic nervous system leading to high concentrations of catecholamines in the blood. Again, the edema is of the high-permeability type.

Overinflation of the lung can cause pulmonary edema. This is sometimes seen in the intensive care unit when high levels of positive end-expiratory pressure (PEEP) are used (*see* Chapter 9). Again, the resulting large tensile forces in the alveolar walls resulting from the high lung volume apparently damage the capillary walls.

Heroin overdosage can cause pulmonary edema. The condition is particularly seen in addicts who inject the drug intravenously when it is mixed with various diluents. These diluents might be partly responsible; however, edema can also follow oral ingestion.

Clinical Features of Pulmonary Edema

Many of the typical features were seen in George. Dyspnea is always a prominent symptom; breathing is typically rapid and shallow, probably because of stimulation of the J receptors in the alveolar walls (*see* Chapter 2). Dyspnea is particularly marked on exertion. Orthopnea (increased dyspnea while recumbent) is common. Paroxysmal nocturnal dyspnea (the patient wakes up at night with severe dyspnea and wheezing) and periodic breathing (the breathing waxes and wanes) may occur. Cough is frequent. It is unproductive in the early stages, but in fulminating edema the patient may cough up large quantities of pink foamy fluid, and indeed may drown in his edema fluid. In severe alveolar edema, cyanosis is seen.

On auscultation of the lungs, rales (crackles) on inspiration are heard particularly at the lung bases as a result of fluid in the airways. In severe edema, rhonchi (musical sounds) may also be present; these are caused by turbulence in airways partly obstructed by edema fluid.

The chest radiograph is often very valuable. Severe *alveolar edema* causes blotchy shadowing which is bilateral (Fig. 7–1). Sometimes the opacities are most marked near the hilar regions, giving a so-called bat's wing, or butterfly, appearance. The explanation may be related to the perivascular and peribronchial cuffing that is particularly noticeable around the large vessels in the hilar region (Figs. 7–2 and 7–3). *Interstitial edema* causes subtle changes in the chest radiograph. The most important findings are septal lines, which are short, linear, horizontal markings originating near the pleural surface in the lower zones **(FIGURE 7–5)**. These are caused by edematous interlobular septa. Although these are difficult radiographic signs to interpret, they often constitute one of the few pieces of evidence for interstitial edema.

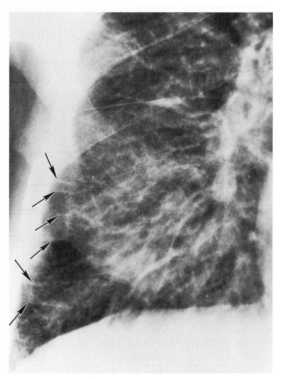

FIGURE 7–5. Septal lines in a patient with marked pulmonary interstitial edema. These short, linear horizontal markings near the pleural surface *(arrows)* are frequently difficult to interpret.

Pulmonary Function

Pulmonary function tests are not normally carried out on patients with pulmonary edema, because they are not required, and the patients are usually so sick.

Gas Exchange

Gas exchange is often severely impaired when alveolar edema is present. The chief cause is complete obstruction of ventilation to some regions of the lung by the edema fluid (Fig. 7–4). This is known as shunt. It could be argued that this is simply an extreme mismatch of ventilation and blood flow, as depicted in Figure 3–18B. However, it is useful to distinguish shunt as a cause of hypoxemia from other patterns of ventilation-perfusion inequality because of the different behavior of the arterial P_{O_2} when 100% O_2 is breathed when a shunt is present (see below).

Shunt

Shunt refers to blood that finds its way into the arterial system without going through ventilated areas of lung. Even in the normal lung, there is a small amount of shunt because some of the blood from the bronchial arteries is collected by the pulmonary veins after it has perfused the bronchi and its O_2 concentration has been partly depleted. Another source is a small amount of coronary venous blood that drains directly into the cavity of the left ventricle through the Thebesian veins. (Most of the venous drainage from the myocardium enters the right atrium via the coronary sinus.) The effect of the addition of this poorly oxygenated blood is to depress the arterial P_{O_2}. However, in normal subjects the reduction of arterial P_{O_2} by these shunts is only about 5 mm Hg, which is barely measurable. By contrast, in patients like George, severe arterial hypoxemia may develop as a result of shunt. This mechanism is also very important in children with cyanotic congenital heart disease, where there is a direct addition of venous blood to arterial blood across a defect between the right and left sides of the heart.

When shunt is caused by the addition of mixed venous blood to blood draining from the capillaries, as in the case of George, it is possible to calculate the proportion of shunt flow (**FIGURE 7–6**). To do this we use a simple mixing

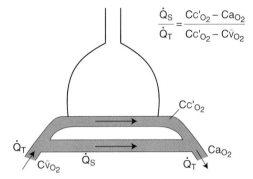

$$\frac{\dot{Q}_S}{\dot{Q}_T} = \frac{Cc'_{O_2} - Ca_{O_2}}{Cc'_{O_2} - C\bar{v}_{O_2}}$$

FIGURE 7–6. Measurement of shunt flow. The oxygen carried in the arterial blood equals the sum of the oxygen carried in the capillary blood together with that in the shunted blood.

equation. The total amount of O_2 leaving the system is the total blood flow $\dot{Q}_T$ multiplied by the O_2 concentration of the arterial blood Ca_{O_2}, or $\dot{Q}_T \times Ca_{O_2}$. This must equal the sum of the amounts of O_2 in the shunted blood, $\dot{Q}_S \times C\bar{v}_{O_2}$, and end-capillary blood, $(\dot{Q}_T - \dot{Q}_S) \times Cc'_{O_2}$. Therefore:

$$\dot{Q}_T \times Ca_{O_2} = \dot{Q}_S \times C\bar{v}_{O_2} + (\dot{Q}_T - \dot{Q}_S) \times Cc'_{O_2}$$

Rearranging, this gives:

$$\frac{\dot{Q}_S}{\dot{Q}_T} = \frac{Cc'_{O_2} - Ca_{O_2}}{Cc'_{O_2} - C\bar{v}_{O_2}}$$

When the lung is normal, as it often is in a patient with cyanotic congenital heart disease, for example, the O_2 concentration of end-capillary blood can be calculated from the alveolar P_{O_2} and the O_2 dissociation curve (see Fig. 1–14).

When the shunt is caused by blood that does not have the same O_2 concentration as mixed venous blood, it is generally not possible to calculate its true magnitude. However, it is often useful to calculate an "as if" shunt, that is, what the shunt would be if the observed depression of arterial O_2 concentration was caused by the addition of mixed venous blood.

An important feature of a shunt is that the hypoxemia cannot be abolished by giving the patient 100% O_2 to breathe. This is because the shunted blood that bypasses ventilated alveoli is never exposed to the high alveolar P_{O_2}, with the result that it continues to depress the arterial P_{O_2}. However, some elevation of the arterial P_{O_2} occurs because of the O_2 added to the capillary blood of ventilated lung. Most of this added O_2 is in the dissolved form, rather than combined with hemoglobin, because the blood that is perfusing ventilated alveoli is nearly fully saturated when air is breathed. Giving a patient 100% O_2 to breathe is a very sensitive measurement of shunt. This is because when the P_{O_2} is high, a small depression of arterial O_2 concentration causes a relatively large fall in arterial P_{O_2}, due to the almost flat slope of the O_2 dissociation curve in this region (FIGURE 7–7). In fact, the slope of the graph of O_2 concentration against P_{O_2} at high P_{O_2} values is solely attributable to the dissolved O_2. Therefore the slope is $0.003 \text{ ml} \cdot \text{dl}^{-1} \cdot \text{mm Hg } P_{O_2}^{-1}$. When George was given 100% O_2 by mouthpiece for 5 min, his arterial P_{O_2} rose to only 200 mm Hg, which was well below the expected value of more than 600 mm Hg, confirming the presence of a large shunt.

A shunt does not usually result in a raised P_{CO_2} in arterial blood, even though the shunted blood is relatively rich in CO_2. This was the case with George, whose arterial blood gas sample showed an arterial P_{CO_2} of 35 mm Hg. One reason why the arterial P_{CO_2} does not rise is that the chemoreceptors sense any elevation of arterial P_{CO_2}, and they respond by increasing the ventilation. In George, stimulation of the J receptors by the edema also probably stimulated breathing. Finally, his hypoxemia may increase respiratory drive.

Although shunt is probably the most important mechanism of hypoxemia in the case of George, lung units with low ventilation-perfusion ratios also contribute to hypoxemia. These either lie behind airways partly obstructed by edema fluid, or are units where the ventilation is reduced by their proximity to nonventilating edematous alveoli. Such units are particularly liable to collapse when a patient is given oxygen to breathe (see Chapter 9), but oxygen therapy is often essential to relieve the hypoxemia and was certainly indicated for George.

Another factor that often exaggerates the arterial hypoxemia in patients like George is a low cardiac output. This occurs because the left ventricle is damaged by the infarct, and its ability to eject blood during systole is impaired. A reduction in cardiac output results in a fall in the P_{O_2} of mixed venous blood, because the peripheral tissues continue to extract oxygen at the same rate (or nearly so), and the Fick equation therefore implies that the arterial-venous O_2 difference is increased. A fall in the P_{O_2} of mixed venous blood reduces the arterial P_{O_2} in the presence of shunt or ventilation-perfusion inequality, as may be deduced from Figures 3–18 and 3–21.

Note that George's arterial pH is slightly reduced at 7.35, even though we would expect it to rise slightly because of his reduced arterial

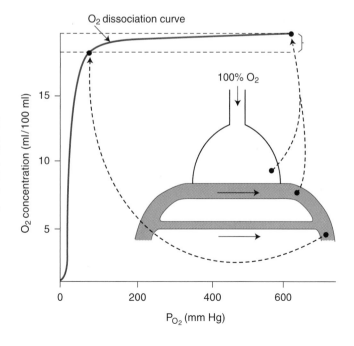

FIGURE 7–7. Depression of the arterial P_{O_2} by shunt during 100% O_2 breathing. The addition of a small amount of shunted blood with its low O_2 concentration greatly reduces the P_{O_2} of arterial blood. This is because the O_2 dissociation curve is so nearly flat when the P_{O_2} is very high.

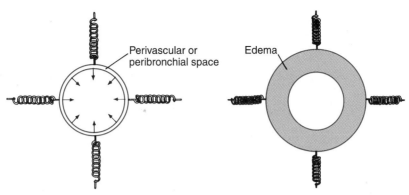

FIGURE 7–8. Diagram showing how interstitial edema in the perivascular or peribronchial region can reduce the caliber of an airway or blood vessel. The cuff of edema isolates the structure from the radial traction of the surrounding parenchyma.

P_{CO_2}. The reason is the addition of lactic acid to his blood by peripheral tissues that are inadequately perfused because of the low cardiac output. Indeed, part of the increase in ventilation resulting in the decreased arterial P_{CO_2} may be stimulation of the peripheral chemoreceptors by the slightly increased H^+ concentration.

While alveolar edema often causes severe hypoxemia, pure interstitial edema (Fig. 7–2) may have minimal effects on gas exchange.

Pulmonary Mechanics

Pulmonary mechanics are altered in alveolar edema. The edema fluid reduces the distensibility of the lung and moves the pressure-volume curve downward and to the right (compare with Fig. 4–4). An important factor in this is the alveolar flooding, which causes a reduction in volume of the affected lung units as a result of surface tension forces, and reduces their participation in the pressure-volume curve. In addition, interstitial edema may stiffen the lung by interfering with its elastic properties, although it is difficult to obtain clear evidence on this. Edematous lungs often require abnormally large expanding pressures during mechanical ventilation and tend to collapse to abnormally small volumes when not actively inflated (*see* Chapter 9).

Airway resistance is typically increased, especially if some of the larger airways contain edema fluid. Reflex bronchoconstriction after stimulation of irritant receptors in the bronchial walls may also play a role. It is possible that even in the absence of alveolar edema, interstitial edema increases the resistance of small airways as a result of their peribronchial cuff (Fig. 7–2). This can be thought of as actually compressing the small airways or, at least, isolating them from the normal traction of the surrounding parenchyma **(FIGURE 7–8)**. There is some evidence that this mechanism promotes airway closure in dependent lung regions and thus causes their intermittent ventilation. The same mechanism is responsible for the increase of pulmonary vascular resistance when interstitial edema is present.

Control of Ventilation

Control of ventilation is often altered by pulmonary edema. As we have seen, George presented to the emergency department with rapid, shallow breathing. This was probably partly caused by stimulation of J receptors in the alveolar walls. Other stimuli include a reduced P_{O_2} and perhaps an increased H^+ concentration in the arterial blood, as in the case of George.

Questions

**For each question, choose the one best answer.
(For answers, see p. 150.)**

1. **Clinical features of alveolar pulmonary edema typically include all of the following EXCEPT:**
   A. Dyspnea
   B. Pleuritic pain
   C. Cough
   D. Crackles at the lung bases
   E. Radiographic changes

2. **All of the following statements about the blood-gas barrier in the normal lung are true EXCEPT:**
   A. Fluid can drain through the interstitium of the thick side of the blood-gas barrier.
   B. The alveolar epithelium has a high permeability for water.
   C. The strength of the barrier on the thin side is mainly attributable to the basement membranes.
   D. Some protein normally crosses the capillary endothelium.
   E. Water is actively pumped out of the alveolar spaces by alveolar epithelial cells.

3. **Interstitial pulmonary edema (in the absence of alveolar edema) typically results in:**
   A. Septal lines on the chest radiograph
   B. Increased lung compliance
   C. Reduced lymph flow from the lungs
   D. Severe hypoxemia
   E. Fluffy shadowing on the chest radiograph

4. **All of the following are true of fluid movement out of pulmonary capillaries EXCEPT:**
   A. Any rise in pulmonary capillary pressure increases lymph flow.
   B. Mean left atrial pressure can exceed pulmonary capillary pressure at mid-lung during severe exercise.
   C. The amount of fluid in the interstitium of the lung increases during heavy exercise.

   D. Lymph draining from the lung contains albumin.
   E. The reflection coefficient of the capillary endothelium is less than 1.

5. **When pulmonary capillary pressure rises, which of the following tends to reduce the formation of edema?**
   A. Reduction of colloid osmotic pressure of the interstitial fluid
   B. Increase in hydrostatic pressure of the interstitial fluid
   C. Increase in reflection coefficient of the capillary endothelium
   D. A and B
   E. None of the above

6. **The following statements are true about high-altitude pulmonary edema EXCEPT:**
   A. Pulmonary wedge pressure is normal.
   B. Pulmonary artery pressure is high.
   C. Edema fluid in the alveoli has a high protein concentration.
   D. Hypoxic pulmonary vasoconstriction may be uneven.
   E. The best immediate treatment is to give diuretics.

7. **A patient has an arteriovenous fistula in an otherwise normal lung. This results in a shunt from a small pulmonary artery to a pulmonary vein. The following measurements were obtained: O_2 concentration in arterial blood 19 ml · dl^{-1}, O_2 concentration in mixed venous blood 15 ml · dl^{-1}, alveolar P_{O_2} 100 mm Hg, and hemoglobin concentration 15.1 g · dl^{-1}. The shunt, as a percentage of cardiac output, is approximately:**
   A. 5
   B. 10
   C. 15
   D. 20
   E. 30

8. **A patient has arterial hypoxemia while breathing air. If the patient is given 100% O_2 via a mouthpiece, all of the following statements are true about the rise in arterial P_{O_2} EXCEPT:**
   A. If the hypoxemia is caused by a shunt, there will be no increase.
   B. If the hypoxemia is caused by hypoventilation, the P_{O_2} will exceed 500 mm Hg.
   C. If the hypoxemia is caused by $\dot{V}_A/\dot{Q}$ inequality, the arterial P_{O_2} will exceed 300 mm Hg.
   D. If the hypoxemia is caused by diffusion impairment, there will be a large rise in arterial P_{O_2}.
   E. If the patient has areas of very low $\dot{V}_A/\dot{Q}$, these may be converted into a shunt.

Chapter 8

Coal Workers' Pneumoconiosis

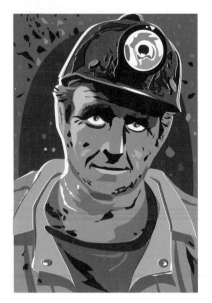

☐ Harry is a 60-year-old, retired coal miner whose chief complaints are shortness of breath and cough. He spent more than 30 years in the mines, much of this time at the coal face. He has smoked one to two packs of cigarettes a day for most of his life. A chest radiograph showed the changes of simple pneumoconiosis, and he is receiving disability payments. In this chapter, we discuss the deposition and clearance of inhaled aerosol and some of the diseases caused by inhaled dusts. The role of cigarette smoking in Harry's disease is also considered.

☐ CLINICAL FINDINGS

History

Harry is a 60-year-old, retired coal miner whose chief complaints are shortness of breath, fatigue, and productive cough. He started working in the mines at 17 years of age and spent much of his life working at the coal face. Over the past 12 years, he has become increasingly short of breath, which he notices particularly if he climbs stairs. However, he can walk on level ground as far as he wants to without pausing for breath. His cough is worst in the morning on waking. The cough is occasionally productive of sputum, particularly in the winter when he gets a cold that "goes to his chest." He has smoked cigarettes since the age of 15, at the rate of one to two packs per day. The mining company arranged for periodical chest radiographs throughout Harry's working life, and 10 years ago he was told that he had a mild case of "black lung" (coal workers' pneumoconiosis). Since then, he has been receiving disability payments. He has not had chest pain or swelling of the ankles. Both his father and grandfather were coal miners, and both were told that mining had affected their lungs.

Physical Examination

The patient did not appear to be short of breath at rest. Vital signs were normal. The only positive findings were that the chest appeared to be slightly overinflated, and occasional rhonchi (musical sounds) were heard by auscultation.

Investigations

Hemoglobin and blood count were normal. A chest radiograph (FIGURE 8–1) showed fine micronodular mottling in both lung fields. No areas of localized fibrosis were seen.

Pulmonary Function Tests

TABLE 8–1 shows that the results of the pulmonary function tests were mildly abnormal. There were small reductions in FEV_1, FVC, and FEV/FVC%. Residual volume was slightly in-

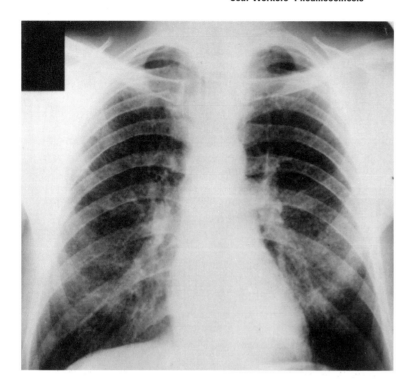

FIGURE 8–1. Chest radiograph showing simple coal workers' pneumoconiosis. The original film showed a delicate micronodular mottling, but this is difficult to reproduce.

TABLE 8–1
Pulmonary Function Tests

Lung Volumes	Observed	Predicted
VC (liters)	4.7	4.8
TLC (liters)	7.3	6.9
FRC (liters)	4.0	3.7
RV (liters)	2.7	2.3
Forced Expiration		
FEV_1 (liters)	3.2	3.8
FVC (liters)	4.6	4.8
FEV/FVC%	69	78
$FEF_{25-75\%}$ ($l \cdot sec^{-1}$)	3.2	3.6
Arterial Blood Gases		
P_{O_2} (mm Hg)	78	85
P_{CO_2} (mm Hg)	39	40
pH	7.41	7.40
Diffusing Capacity for CO		
($ml \cdot min^{-1} \cdot mm\ Hg^{-1}$)	26	28

creased. The arterial blood gases showed a small reduction in P_{O_2}, but the P_{CO_2} and pH were normal.

Diagnosis

Simple coal workers' pneumoconiosis and chronic bronchitis.

Treatment and Progress

The patient was strongly advised to stop smoking, but he found this impossible to do. Exacerbations of his bronchitis during the winter responded to antibiotics. Since the patient was not severely disabled, he did not pursue further treatment.

☐ PATHOGENESIS

Harry's story is (or was) a common one in the coal mining industry. Dust suppression procedures have now greatly reduced the incidence of these conditions. The diagnosis of simple pneumoconiosis was based on the appearance on the chest radiograph (Fig. 8–1), and was sufficient to classify Harry as medically disabled. However, it is not clear to what extent the symptoms, signs, and mild reduction in pulmonary function in a patient like this can be attributed to his pneumoconiosis on the one hand, or his chronic bronchitis and possibly emphysema on the other. Harry has a long smoking history, and it is difficult to be sure to what extent his coal

mining has been a factor in his present clinical presentation.

Harry's condition gives us the opportunity of discussing the consequences of inhaling atmospheric pollutants. These are important, not only in the specific pneumoconioses such as coal workers' pneumoconiosis, silicosis (caused by inhaled silica dust), asbestos-related diseases, and byssinosis (inhaled cotton dust), but atmospheric pollutants are also significant factors in the etiology of other diseases, such as chronic bronchitis, emphysema, asthma, and bronchial carcinoma.

☐ ATMOSPHERIC POLLUTANTS

Types of Pollutants

Carbon Monoxide

This is the largest pollutant by weight in the United States (**FIGURE 8–2A**). It is produced by the incomplete combustion of carbon in fuels, chiefly in the automobile engine (Fig. 8–2B). The main hazard of carbon monoxide is its ability to tie up hemoglobin; because carbon monoxide has about 240 times the affinity of oxygen, it competes successfully with this gas (see discussion in Chapter 1). A commuter using a busy urban freeway may have 5 to 10% of his hemoglobin bound to carbon monoxide, particularly if he is a cigarette smoker. There is evidence that this can impair mental skills. The emission of carbon monoxide and other pollutants by automobile engines can be reduced by

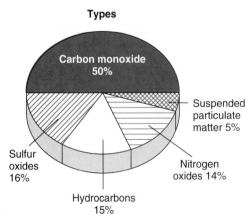 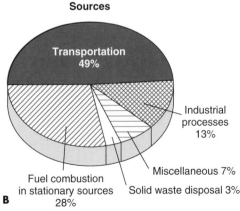

FIGURE 8–2. Air pollutants (by weight) in the United States. Transportation sources, especially automobiles, account for the largest amounts of pollutants. (Data are from the Environmental Protection Agency.)

installing a catalytic converter that processes the exhaust gases.

Nitrogen Oxides

These are produced when fossil fuels (coal, oil) are burned at high temperatures in power stations and automobiles. These gases cause inflammation of the eyes and upper respiratory tract during smoggy conditions. At high concentrations, they can cause acute tracheitis, acute bronchitis, and pulmonary edema. The yellow haze of smog is caused by these gases.

Sulfur Oxides

These are corrosive, poisonous gases produced when sulfur-containing fuels are burned, chiefly by power stations. These gases cause inflammation of the mucous membranes, eyes, upper respiratory tract, and bronchial mucosa. Short-term exposure to high concentrations causes pulmonary edema. Long-term exposure to lower levels results in chronic bronchitis in experimental animals. The best way to reduce emissions of sulfur oxides is to use low-sulfur fuels, but these are more expensive.

Hydrocarbons

Hydrocarbons, like carbon monoxide, represent unburned, wasted fuel. They are not toxic at concentrations normally found in the atmosphere. However, they are hazardous because they form photochemical oxidants under the influence of sunlight (see below).

Particulate Matter

These include particles with a wide range of sizes, up to visible smoke and soot. Major sources are power stations and industrial plants. Often their emission can be reduced by processing the waste air stream by filtering or scrubbing, although removing the smallest particles is usually expensive. The pneumoconioses are caused by special particulates, such as coal dust, silica dust, asbestos particles, and cotton dust. In very dusty environments, such as the coal face in a mine, water sprays and special tools are now used to reduce the dust concentration in the air. This has led to a striking decrease in the incidence of coal workers' pneumoconiosis.

Photochemical Oxidants

These include ozone and other substances, such as peroxyacyl nitrates, aldehydes, and acrolein. They are not primary emissions, but are produced by the action of sunlight on hydrocarbons and nitrogen oxides. They cause inflammation of the eyes and respiratory tract, damage to vegetation, and offensive odors. In higher concentrations, ozone causes pulmonary edema. These oxidants contribute to the thick haze of smog.

The concentration of atmospheric pollutants is often greatly increased by a temperature inversion, that is, a low layer of cold air below warmer air. This prevents the normal escape of warm surface air, with its pollutants, to the upper atmosphere. The deleterious effects of a temperature inversion are particularly significant in a low-lying area surrounded by hills, such as the Los Angeles basin.

Cigarette Smoke

This is one of the most important pollutants in practice because it is inhaled by devotees in concentrations many times greater than are pollutants in the atmosphere. It includes approximately 4% carbon monoxide, enough to raise the carboxyhemoglobin level in a smoker's blood to 10%. This percentage is sufficient to impair exercise and mental performance. The smoke also contains the alkaloid nicotine which stimulates the autonomic nervous system, causing tachycardia, hypertension, and sweating. Aromatic hydrocarbons and other substances, loosely called "tars," are apparently responsible for the high risk of bronchial carcinoma in cigarette smokers. For example, a male who smokes 35 cigarettes per day has 40 times the risk of a nonsmoker. Increased risks of chronic bronchitis and emphysema, and of coronary heart disease, are also well documented. A single cigarette causes a marked increase in airway resistance in many smokers and nonsmokers.

☐ DEPOSITION OF AEROSOLS IN THE LUNG

The term "aerosol" refers to a collection of particles that remains airborne for a substantial amount of time. Many pollutants exist in this form, and their pattern of deposition in the lung depends chiefly on their size. The properties of aerosols are also important in understanding the distribution of inhaled bronchodilators. Three mechanisms of deposition are recognized.

Impaction

This refers to the tendency of the largest inspired particles to fail to turn the corners of the respiratory tract. As a result, many particles impinge on the mucous surfaces of the nose and pharynx (**FIGURE 8–3A**) and also on the bifurca-

tions of the large airways. Once a particle strikes a wet surface, it is trapped and not subsequently released. The nose is remarkably efficient at removing the largest particles by this mechanism; almost all particles greater than 20 μm in diameter and approximately 95% of particles 5 μm in diameter are filtered by the nose during resting breathing. **FIGURE 8–4** shows that most of the deposition of particles larger than 3 μm in diameter occurs in the nasopharynx during nose breathing.

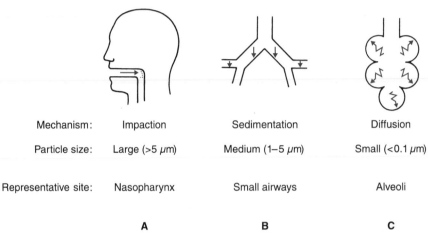

Mechanism:	Impaction	Sedimentation	Diffusion
Particle size:	Large (>5 μm)	Medium (1–5 μm)	Small (<0.1 μm)
Representative site:	Nasopharynx	Small airways	Alveoli

    A   **B**   **C**

FIGURE 8–3. Deposition of aerosols in the lung. The term "representative site" does not mean that these are the only sites where this form of deposition occurs. For example, impaction also occurs in medium-sized bronchi, and diffusion also occurs in the large and small airways. (See text for details.)

FIGURE 8–4. Site of deposition of aerosols in the lung. The largest particles remain in the nasopharynx, but the smallest particles can penetrate to the alveoli.

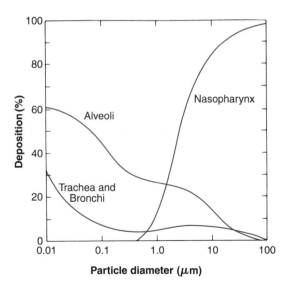

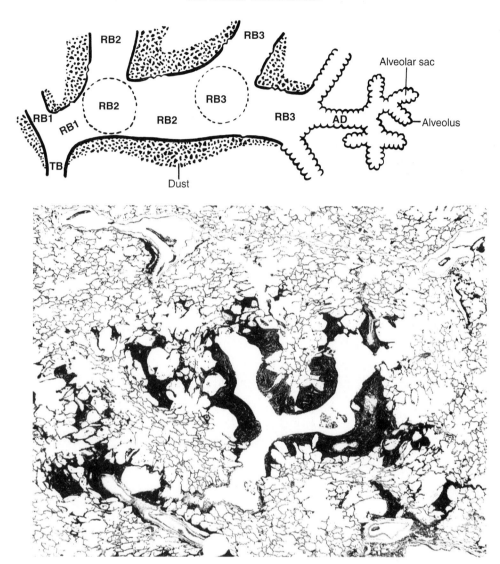

FIGURE 8–5. Microscopic section of lung from a coal miner, showing accumulations of coal dust around the respiratory bronchioles. These airways also show some dilation.

Sedimentation

This refers to the gradual settling of particles because of their weight (Fig. 8–3B). It is particularly important for medium-sized particles (1 to 5 µm), because the largest particles are removed by impaction, and the smaller particles settle so slowly. Deposition by sedimentation occurs extensively in the small airways, including the terminal and respiratory bronchioles. The chief reason is simply that the dimensions of those airways are so small, and therefore the particles have a shorter distance to

fall. Particles, unlike gases, are not able to diffuse from the respiratory bronchioles to the alveoli because of their negligibly small diffusion rate (see discussion of Fig. 4–8).

The importance of sedimentation in the region of the terminal and respiratory bronchioles can be underlined if we look at a microscopic section of lung from a coal miner like Harry **(FIGURE 8–5)**. Note the accumulations of dust around the terminal and respiratory bronchioles. This is the pathological basis of the micronodular mottling seen in the chest radiograph in simple pneumoconiosis (Fig. 8–1). It should be added that the retention of dust depends not only on its deposition, but also its clearance, and it is possible that some of this dust was transported from peripheral alveoli. Nevertheless, Figure 8–5 is a graphic reminder of the vulnerability of the terminal and respiratory bronchioles. It is also likely that some of the earliest changes in chronic bronchitis are secondary to the deposition of atmospheric pollutants (including tobacco smoke particles) in the small airways.

Diffusion

This is the random movement of particles as a result of their continuous bombardment by gas molecules (Fig. 8–3C). It occurs to a significant extent only in the smallest particles, less than 0.1 µm in diameter. Deposition by diffusion chiefly takes place in the small airways and alveoli, where the distances to the wall are the smallest. However, some deposition by this mechanism also occurs in the larger airways.

Many inhaled particles are not deposited at all, but are exhaled with the next breath. In fact, only some 30% of 0.5 µm particles may be left in the lung during normal resting breathing. These particles are too small to impact or sediment to a large extent. In addition, they are too large to diffuse significantly. As a result, they do not move from the terminal and respiratory bronchioles to the alveoli by diffusion, which is the normal mode of gas movement in this region. Some particles may become larger during inspiration by aggregation or by absorbing water.

The pattern of ventilation affects the amount of aerosol deposition. Slow, deep breaths increase the penetration into the lung and thus increase the amount of dust deposited by sedimentation and diffusion. Exercise results in higher rates of airflow and particularly increases deposition by impaction. In general, deposition of dust is proportional to the ventilation during exercise. Therefore, in the case of a coal miner like Harry, who was doing hard physical work in the vicinity of the coal face where dust concentrations were high, the risks were increased.

☐ CLEARANCE OF DEPOSITED PARTICLES

Fortunately, the lung is efficient at removing particles that are deposited within it. Two distinct clearance mechanisms exist: the muco-ciliary system and the alveolar macrophages (FIGURE 8–6).

Mucociliary System

Mucus is produced by two sources. Bronchial seromucous glands situated deep in the bronchial walls (see Figs. 3–4, 3–5, and FIGURE 8–7) are the first source. Both mucus-producing and serous-producing cells are present, and ducts lead the mucus to the airway surface. Goblet cells, which form part of the bronchial epithelium, are the second source.

The normal mucous film is approximately 5 to 10 µm thick and has two layers (Fig. 8–7). The superficial gel layer is relatively tenacious and viscous. As a result, it is efficient at trapping deposited particles. The deeper sol layer is less viscous and therefore allows the cilia to beat within it easily. It is likely that the abnormal retention of secretions that occurs in some diseases is caused by changes in the composition

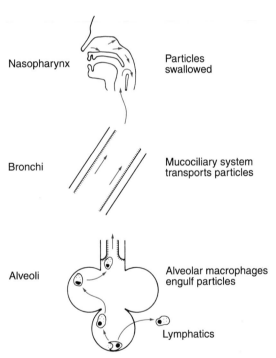

FIGURE 8–6. Clearance of inhaled particles from the lung. Particles that deposit on the surface of the airways are transported by the mucociliary escalator and swallowed. Particles that reach the alveoli are engulfed by macrophages, which either migrate to the ciliary surface or escape via the lymphatics.

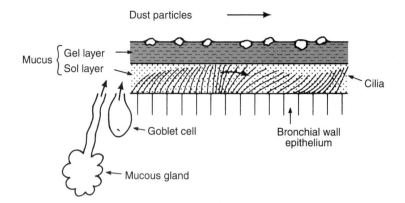

FIGURE 8–7. Mucociliary escalator. The mucous film consists of a superficial gel layer that traps inhaled particles and a deeper sol layer. It is propelled by cilia.

of the mucus, with the result that it cannot be propelled easily by the cilia. An example is asthma in which, as described in Chapter 4, the mucus is thick, tenacious, and slow moving and many of the airways are occluded by mucous plugs.

The mucus contains immunoglobulin A (IgA), which is derived from plasma cells and lymphoid tissue. This humoral factor is an important defense against foreign proteins, bacteria, and viruses.

The cilia are 5 to 7 μm in length and beat in a synchronized fashion between 1000 and 1500 times per minute. During the forward stroke, the tips of the cilia apparently come in contact with the gel layer, thus propelling it. However, during the recovery phase, the cilia are bent so much that they move entirely within the sol layer, where the resistance is less.

The mucous blanket moves up at about 1 mm · min^{-1} in small peripheral airways and as fast at 2 cm · min^{-1} in the trachea; eventually, the particles reach the level of the pharynx where they are swallowed. The clearance of a healthy bronchial mucosa is essentially complete in less than 24 hours. In very dusty environments, mucous secretion may be increased so much that cough and expectoration assist in the clearance.

The normal operation of the mucociliary system is affected by pollution or disease. The cilia can be paralyzed by the inhalation of toxic gases, such as oxides of sulfur and nitrogen, and perhaps by tobacco smoke. In acute inflammation of the respiratory tract, the bronchial epithelium may be denuded. Changes in the character of the mucus may occur with infection, thus making it difficult for cilia to transport it. Mucous plugging of bronchi in asthma has

already been referred to. In chronic infections, such as bronchiectasis or chronic bronchitis, the volume of secretions may be so great that the ciliary transport system is overloaded.

Alveolar Macrophages

The mucociliary system stops short of the alveoli, and particles deposited there are engulfed by macrophages. These amoeboid cells roam around the surface of the alveoli. When they phagocytose foreign particles, they either migrate to the small airways where they load onto the mucociliary escalator (Fig. 8–6) or they leave the lung in the lymphatics or possibly the blood. When the dust burden is large, or the dust particles are toxic, some of the macrophages migrate through the walls of the respiratory bronchioles and dump their dust there. Figure 8–5 shows accumulations of coal dust around the respiratory bronchioles in the lungs of a coal miner. If the dust is toxic, as is silica dust, a fibrous reaction is stimulated in this region.

The macrophages not only transport bacteria out of the lung, but also kill them in situ by means of the lysozymes they contain. As a consequence, the alveoli quickly become sterile, although it takes some time for the dead organisms to be cleared from the lung. Immunological mechanisms are also important in the antibacterial action of macrophages.

Normal macrophage activity can be impaired by various factors such as cigarette smoke, oxidant gases such as ozone, alveolar hypoxia, radiation, the administration of corticosteroids, and the ingestion of alcohol. Macrophages that engulf particles of silica are often killed by this toxic material.

☐ PNEUMOCONIOSES AND RELATED CONDITIONS

Strictly, the term "pneumoconiosis" refers to parenchymal lung disease caused by inorganic dust inhalation.

Coal Workers' Pneumoconiosis

Some features of this were referred to when we discussed Harry's disease. He has simple pneumoconiosis, which is characterized by aggregations of coal particles around terminal and respiratory bronchioles, with some dilatation of these small airways (Fig. 8–5). There is also an advanced form of the disease, known as *progressive massive fibrosis*. Here, the lung contains condensed masses of black fibrous tissue infiltrated with dust **(FIGURE 8–8)**. Only a small fraction of coal miners exposed to heavy dust concentrations develop progressive massive fibrosis.

As already mentioned, simple pneumoconiosis probably causes little disability despite its radiographic appearances. The dyspnea and cough that often accompany the disease are closely related to the smoking history of the miner and are probably caused by associated chronic bronchitis and emphysema. By contrast, progressive massive fibrosis usually causes increasing dyspnea and may terminate in respiratory failure.

We have seen that the chest radiograph in simple pneumoconiosis shows a delicate micronodular mottling (Fig. 8–1), and various stages in the advance of the disease are recognized, depending on the pattern of the shadows. Progressive massive fibrosis results in large, irregular dense opacities, often surrounded by abnormally translucent lung. Figure 8–8 shows an example which was unusual in that simple pulmonary function tests were within normal limits for the patient's age despite the striking extent of disease.

Simple pneumoconiosis usually causes only minor changes in pulmonary function. Sometimes a small reduction in FEV, rise in residual volume, and fall in arterial P_{O_2} are seen, but it is often difficult to know whether these changes are caused by associated chronic bronchitis and emphysema, as in the case of Harry. Progressive massive fibrosis typically causes a mixed obstructive and restrictive pattern. Distortion of the airways results in irreversible obstructive

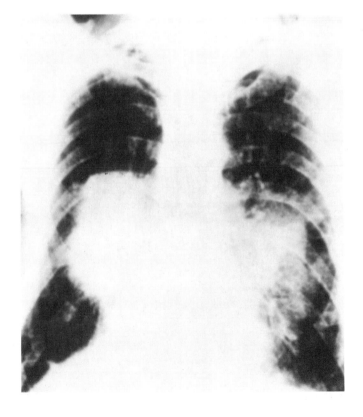

FIGURE 8–8. Chest radiograph of an 81-year-old coal miner with advanced bilateral progressive massive fibrosis. Astonishingly, simple pulmonary function tests were within normal limits for his age. For example, his arterial P_{O_2} and P_{CO_2} were 79 and 36 mm Hg, respectively.

changes, and the large masses of fibrous tissue reduce the useful volume of the lung. Increasing hypoxemia, cor pulmonale, and terminal respiratory failure may occur.

Silicosis

This pneumoconiosis is caused by the inhalation of silica (SiO_2) during quarrying, mining, or sandblasting. Whereas coal dust is virtually inert, silica particles are toxic and provoke a severe fibrous reaction in the lung. Silicotic nodules, composed of concentric whorls of dense collagen fibers, are found around respiratory bronchioles, inside alveoli, and along the lymphatics. Silica particles can be seen in the nodules.

Mild forms of the disease may cause no symptoms, although the chest radiograph shows fine nodular markings. Advanced disease results in cough and severe dyspnea, especially on exercise. The radiograph sometimes shows streaks of fibrous tissue, and progressive massive fibrosis may develop. The disease may progress long after exposure to the dust has ceased, and there is an increased risk of pulmonary tuberculosis.

The changes in pulmonary function are similar to those seen in coal workers' pneumoconiosis but are often more severe. In advanced disease, generalized interstitial fibrosis may develop with a restrictive type of defect, severe dyspnea and hypoxemia on exercise, and a reduced diffusing capacity (*see* Chapter 5).

Asbestos-Related Diseases

Asbestos is a naturally occurring fibrous mineral silicate that is used in a variety of industrial applications, including heat insulation, pipe lagging, roofing materials, and brake linings. Asbestos fibers are long and thin, and it is possible that the resulting aerodynamic characteristics allow them to penetrate far into the lung. When deposited in the lung, they may become encased in proteinaceous material. If they are coughed up in the sputum, they have a very distinctive appearance.

Three health hazards are recognized:

1. Diffuse interstitial fibrosis (asbestosis) may gradually occur after heavy exposure (*see* Chapter 5). There is progressive dyspnea (especially on exercise), weakness, and finger clubbing. On auscultation, there may be fine basal crepitations. The chest radiograph shows haziness or mottling. Pulmonary function tests in advanced disease reveal a typical restrictive pattern with reduction of all lung volumes and lung compliance. A fall in diffusing capacity occurs relatively early in the disease.

2. Bronchial carcinoma is a common complication. Cigarette smoking is often an aggravating factor.

3. Pleural disease may occur after trivial exposure (e.g., in a person who washes the clothes of an asbestos worker). Pleural thickening and plaques are common but usually harmless. However, malignant mesothelioma may develop as much as 40 years after light exposure. It causes progressive restriction of chest movement, severe chest pain, and a rapid downhill course.

Other Pneumoconioses

A variety of other dusts cause simple pneumoconiosis. Examples include iron and its oxides which cause siderosis and result in a striking, mottled radiographic appearance. Antimony and tin are other culprits. Beryllium exposure results in granulomatous lesions of acute or chronic types. The latter results in interstitial fibrosis with its typical restrictive pattern of dysfunction. The disease is now much less common than it was, as a result of the strict control of beryllium in industry.

Byssinosis

Some inhaled organic dusts cause airway reactions rather than alveolar reactions as is the case with most of the pneumoconioses. A good example is byssinosis, which follows exposure to cotton dust, especially in the card room where the fibers are initially processed.

The pathogenesis is not fully understood, but it appears that the inhalation of some active component in the bracts (leaves around the stem of the cotton boll) leads to the release of histamine from mast cells in the lung. The resulting bronchoconstriction causes dyspnea and wheezing. A feature of the disease is that the symptoms are worse on entering the mill, especially after a period of absence such as a weekend. For this reason, this disease is sometimes known as "Monday fever." The symptoms include dyspnea, tightness of the chest, wheezing, and an irritating cough. Workers who already have chronic bronchitis or asthma are especially susceptible.

Pulmonary function tests show an obstructive pattern, with reductions in FEV_1, FEV/FVC%, $FEF_{25-75\%}$, and FVC (*see* Chapters 3 and 4). Airway resistance, measured in a body plethysmograph, is increased. In addition, there is an increase in the amount of inequality of ventilation. Typically these abnormalities gradually become worse over the course of a working day, but partial or complete recovery occurs during the night or over the weekend. There is no evidence of parenchyma involvement, and the chest radiograph is normal. However, epidemiological studies show that daily exposure after 20 years or so causes permanent impairment of lung function of the type associated with chronic obstructive pulmonary disease.

Occupational Asthma

Various occupations involve exposure to allergenic organic dusts, and some individuals develop hypersensitivity. These individuals include flour mill workers who are sensitive to the wheat weevil, printers exposed to gum acacia, and workers handling fur or feathers. Toluene diisocyanate (TDI) is a special case because some individuals develop an extreme sensitivity to this substance, which is used in the manufacture of polyurethane products.

Questions For each question, choose the one best answer.
(For answers, see p. 150.)

1. Which of the following atmospheric
   pollutants is present in the highest con-
   centration (by weight) in the United
   States?
   A. Hydrocarbons.
   B. Sulfur oxides.
   C. Nitrogen oxides.
   D. Carbon monoxide.
   E. Ozone.

2. All of the following statements about
   smog are true EXCEPT:
   A. Ozone is produced by the action of sun-
      light on hydrocarbons and nitrogen
      oxides.
   B. The concentration of pollutants at
      ground level can be increased by a tem-
      perature inversion.
   C. The main source of sulfur oxides is the
      automobile engine.
   D. Nitrogen oxides can cause inflammation
      of the upper respiratory tract.
   E. Many particulates can be removed by
      scrubbing flue gases.

3. All of the following statements are true
   about cigarette smoke EXCEPT:
   A. Inhaled smoke can contain more than
      3% carbon monoxide.
   B. Cigarette smokers can have enough car-
      boxyhemoglobin level in their blood to
      impair exercise performance.
   C. Alkaloids in cigarette smoke stimulate
      the autonomic nervous system.
   D. Cigarette smoking increases the risk of
      coronary heart disease.
   E. The concentration of pollutants in ciga-
      rette smoke is less than in the air of a
      large city on a smoggy day.

4. All of the following statements are true
   about the deposition of aerosol in the
   lung EXCEPT:
   A. Most particles greater than 5 μm diame-
      ter are filtered by the nose during resting
      breathing.

   B. Many inhaled particles are deposited in
      the region of the terminal and respira-
      tory bronchioles.
   C. Deposition of particles by sedimentation
      is abolished in astronauts who are
      weightless.
   D. Particles of 0.5 μm diameter diffuse
      almost as fast as gas molecules.
   E. Many particles of 0.5 μm diameter are
      not deposited in the lung but are exhaled
      with the next breath.

5. In a coal miner, the deposition of coal
   dust in the lung will be exaggerated by
   all of the following EXCEPT:
   A. Failure to institute dust suppression
      procedures.
   B. Exercise.
   C. Mining operations that produce dust
      particles less than 10 μm in diameter.
   D. Rapid deep breathing.
   E. Nose breathing, as opposed to mouth
      breathing.

6. All of the following statements about the
   mucociliary escalator in the lung are
   true EXCEPT:
   A. The normal mucous film has two layers.
   B. Trapped particles move more rapidly in
      the trachea than in the peripheral
      airways.
   C. The mucus contains IgA.
   D. The cilia beat about twice a second.
   E. The composition of the mucous film is
      altered in some diseases.

7. All of the following statements about al-
   veolar macrophages are true EXCEPT:
   A. They can be killed by toxic particles.
   B. They engulf foreign matter by phagocy-
      tosis.
   C. Some macrophages leave the lung by
      reaching the mucociliary escalator.
   D. Their normal activity can be inhibited by
      cigarette smoking.
   E. They move by rolling along the surface
      of the alveoli.

8. **All of the following statements are true about asbestos and asbestos-related diseases EXCEPT:**
   A. Asbestos is used for heat insulation.
   B. Macrophages that engulf asbestos fibers are unharmed.
   C. Asbestos can cause diffuse pulmonary interstitial fibrosis.
   D. Pleural plaques can occur long after minor exposure to asbestos.
   E. The shape of the fibers may allow them to penetrate far into the lung.

9. **All of the following statements are true about byssinosis EXCEPT:**
   A. It is caused by inhaled cotton dust.
   B. The major abnormality is bronchoconstriction.
   C. Symptoms are typically worst when exposure to the dust occurs after several days of absence.
   D. Pulmonary function tests show changes in a forced expiration.
   E. The chest radiograph typically shows severe parenchymal disease.

Chapter 9

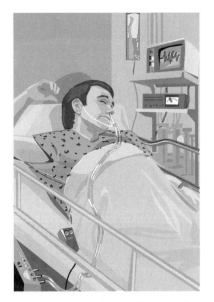

Acute Respiratory Failure

☐ Ivan is a 45-year-old computer programmer who was involved in a serious automobile accident which resulted in fractures of long bones and a blow to his chest. Two days after admission to the hospital, he developed acute respiratory failure with severe hypoxemia and carbon dioxide retention. He was intubated and mechanically ventilated but died on the seventh day after admission. We discuss the pathophysiology of various types of respiratory failure and consider two of the important forms of treatment, oxygen therapy and mechanical ventilation.

☐ CLINICAL FINDINGS

History

Ivan is a 45-year-old computer programmer who was well until 10 days ago, when the car he was driving ran off the road and struck a tree. He sustained fractures of his left humerus and right femur as well as contusion of the lung when his chest hit the steering wheel with considerable force. He was admitted to the hospital, intravenous fluids were administered, the fractures were attended to, and he seemed to be making satisfactory progress. However, on the second day after admission his condition deteriorated. He became very short of breath, and there was some clouding of consciousness.

Physical Examination

When examined on the second day after admission, the patient appeared ill and there was obvious dyspnea and restlessness. Temperature was 38.5°C, blood pressure 125/60 mm Hg, pulse 110 beats · min^{-1}. The left arm and right leg were in plaster. There was no neck vein engorgement. Heart sounds were normal. Auscultation of the chest revealed poor breath sounds and some rales (crackles) in all areas.

Investigations

Hemoglobin and blood cell counts were normal. A chest radiograph **(FIGURE 9–1)** was grossly abnormal, with a bilateral "white out" pattern that was interpreted as showing alveolar exudate or edema in all areas. Arterial blood gases showed a P_{O_2} of 51 mm Hg, P_{CO_2} of 45 mm Hg, and pH 7.31.

Diagnosis

Acute respiratory failure secondary to severe trauma.

Treatment and Progress

The patient was intubated with a cuffed endotracheal tube, and mechanical ventilation was begun with 40% oxygen. A Swan-Ganz catheter was inserted into the right atrium via a peripheral vein to monitor central venous pressure.

The patient initially responded to treatment, and the day after intubation the arterial blood gases were as follows: P_{O_2} 65 mm Hg on 40% O_2, P_{CO_2} 35 mm Hg, pH 7.35. However, despite therapy with antibiotics and steroids, his condition worsened and his arterial P_{O_2} could not be

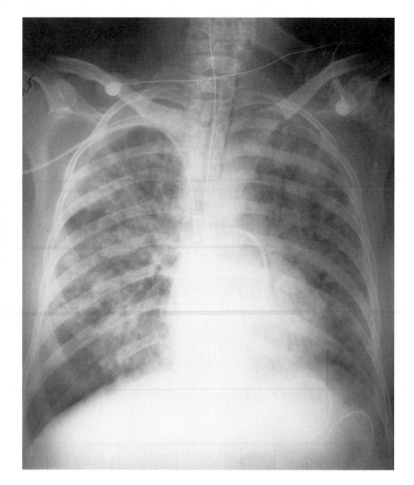

FIGURE 9–1. Chest radiograph of a patient with acute respiratory failure, showing massive filling of alveoli with edema and exudate, especially on the right side. An endotracheal tube and electrocardiogram leads for monitoring can also be seen.

maintained above 50 mm Hg even with 80% O_2. The patient died on the seventh day after admission.

Pathology

A microscopic section of the lung showed red blood cells, cellular debris, and proteinaceous fluid in the alveoli, with patchy atelectasis (FIGURE 9–2). Cellular infiltration of the alveolar walls was also seen.

□ PHYSIOLOGY AND PATHOPHYSIOLOGY

Ivan's clinical presentation and progress provide an example of acute respiratory failure. In this instance, another name for the condition is adult respiratory distress syndrome (ARDS). It re-

sulted from his severe automobile accident. Ivan's disease gives us an opportunity to discuss the various types of respiratory failure, the abnormalities of gas exchange and mechanics, and the principles of two of the chief modes of treatment: oxygen administration and mechanical ventilation.

Pathophysiology of Respiratory Failure

Definition of Respiratory Failure

Respiratory failure is said to occur when the lung fails to oxygenate the arterial blood adequately or fail to prevent CO_2 retention. There is no absolute definition of the levels of arterial P_{O_2} and P_{CO_2} that indicate respiratory failure. However, a P_{O_2} of less than 60 mm Hg, or a P_{CO_2} of more than 50 mm Hg, are numbers that are often quoted. In practice, the significance of such values depends considerably on the history of the patient.

Gas Exchange in Respiratory Failure

The various types of respiratory failure are associated with different degrees of hypoxemia and CO_2 retention. **FIGURE 9–3** shows a so-called O_2–CO_2 diagram, with P_{O_2} on the horizontal axis and P_{CO_2} on the vertical axis. In such a diagram, the alveolar P_{O_2} and P_{CO_2} for a normal respiratory exchange ratio (R) of 0.8 is represented by a straight line IA going up and to the left from the inspired gas point I (i.e., P_{O_2} 149 and P_{CO_2} 0; *see* Fig. 3–18). The normal lung has alveolar P_{O_2} and P_{CO_2} values of 100 and 40 mm Hg, respectively, as indicated by the normal point on the line, and the arterial values are close to these (*see* Fig. 3–18).

Pure hypoventilation moves the arterial P_{O_2} and P_{CO_2} in the direction indicated by arrow A, while pure hyperventilation—as occurred when Bill went to high altitude (*see* Chapter 2)—moves the values in the direction of I. In a steady state, the R value must be approximately 0.8 because this is set by the metabolism of the tissues. In

hypoventilation the increase in P_{CO_2} can be predicted from the alveolar ventilation equation (*see* Chapter 2):

$$P_{CO_2} = \frac{\dot{V}_{CO_2}}{\dot{V}_A} \times K$$

where $\dot{V}_{CO_2}$ is the CO_2 production (this remains essentially constant at rest), and $\dot{V}_A$ is the alveolar ventilation. This pattern occurs in respiratory failure caused by neuromuscular disease, such as poliomyelitis, or by an overdose of a narcotic drug (see below).

Severe ventilation-perfusion ratio inequality with alveolar ventilation inadequate to maintain a normal arterial P_{CO_2} results in movement along a line such as B. The hypoxemia is more severe in relation to the hypercapnia than in the case of pure hyperventilation. Such a pattern frequently occurs in the respiratory failure of chronic obstructive pulmonary disease (COPD), and we saw an example in Chuck in Chapter 3 when he was readmitted to hospital.

Severe interstitial lung disease sometimes results in movement along line C. Here there is increasingly severe hypoxemia, but no CO_2 retention because of the increased ventilation. This pattern may occur in advanced diffuse

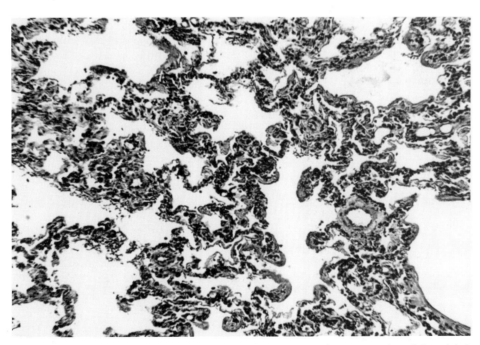

FIGURE 9–2. Histological changes in the adult respiratory distress syndrome (ARDS) as found at autopsy. There is patchy atelectasis, edema, hyaline membranes, and cellular debris in the alveoli.

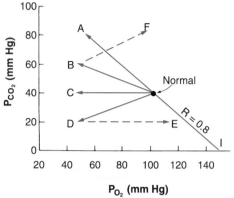

FIGURE 9–3. Patterns of arterial P_{O_2} and P_{CO_2} in different types of respiratory failure. The P_{CO_2} is high in pure hypoventilation (*A*) but may be low in ARDS (*D*). *Broken lines* show the effects of O_2 breathing. (See text for details.)

interstitial lung disease, and we saw an example in Elena (*see* Chapter 5) who developed severe arterial hypoxemia but maintained a normal P_{CO_2}.

In some patients with respiratory failure caused by ARDS the hypoxemia is severe but the arterial P_{CO_2} may be low, as shown by line D. Treatment with added inspired oxygen raises the arterial P_{O_2} but may not affect the P_{CO_2} (D to E), although in some instances it may rise. Oxygen therapy for patients whose respiratory failure is caused by COPD improves the P_{O_2} but frequently causes a rise in P_{CO_2} because of depression of ventilation (B to F). This CO_2 retention especially occurs in patients whose ventilation is strongly stimulated by their hypoxemia (see below).

Hypoxemia of Respiratory Failure

There are four mechanisms of hypoxemia: hypoventilation, diffusion impairment, shunt, and ventilation-perfusion inequality. All these can contribute to the severe hypoxemia of respiratory failure. However, the most important cause by far is ventilation-perfusion inequality (including blood flow through unventilated lung). This was the mechanism in Ivan's case.

Mild hypoxemia causes few physiological changes. Recall that the arterial O_2 saturation is still approximately 90% when the P_{O_2} is only 60

mm Hg at a normal pH (*see* Fig. 1–14). The only abnormalities are a slight impairment of mental performance and visual acuity, and perhaps mild hyperventilation.

However, when the arterial P_{O_2} drops quickly to 40 to 50 mm Hg, deleterious effects are seen in several organ systems. The central nervous system is particularly vulnerable, and the patient often has headache, somnolence, or clouding of consciousness (as in Ivan). The cardiovascular system shows tachycardia and perhaps mild hypertension, partly caused by the release of catecholamines. Signs of heart failure may occur if there is associated coronary artery disease. Renal function is impaired, and sodium retention and proteinuria may be seen. Pulmonary hypertension is common, because of the associated alveolar hypoxia. The hypoxemia of severe respiratory failure affects many organs, and the condition is often regarded as multi-organ failure.

Arterial hypoxemia is dangerous because it causes tissue hypoxia. Organs at the greatest risk include the central nervous system and the myocardium. As discussed in relation to Figure 1–18, a fall in tissue P_{O_2} below a critical level means that aerobic oxidation ceases and anaerobic glycolysis takes over with the formation and release of increasing amounts of lactic acid. Anaerobic glycolysis is a relatively inefficient method of obtaining energy from glucose. Nevertheless, it plays a critical role in maintaining tissue viability in respiratory failure. Release of large amounts of lactic acid into the blood results in metabolic acidosis. Ivan's pH of 7.31 was lower than can be accounted for by the slightly elevated P_{CO_2} of 45 mm Hg. This indicates that there was some associated metabolic acidosis caused by lactate accumulation. We also saw evidence of lactic acidosis in George, who had a myocardial infarct. In that case, the tissue hypoxia was chiefly caused by the reduced blood flow in some regions of the body.

CO_2 Retention in Respiratory Failure

CO_2 retention can be caused by two mechanisms: hypoventilation, and ventilation-perfusion inequality. In pure hypoventilation, the lungs themselves are often normal. Causes include neuromuscular diseases such as poliomyelitis and Guillain-Barré syndrome, drug overdose such as barbiturate poisoning, and a chest wall abnormality such as a crushed chest with broken ribs. The increase in P_{CO_2} can be predicted from the alveolar ventilation equation referred to above. Ventilation-perfusion inequality causes CO_2 retention because a lung with mismatched ventilation and blood flow becomes inefficient at transferring all gases including CO_2 (see discussion in Chapter 3).

An important cause of CO_2 retention in respiratory failure is the injudicious use of O_2 therapy. Many patients with COPD gradually develop severe hypoxemia and some CO_2 retention over a period of months. It is not customary to refer to this situation as respiratory failure because these patients can continue in this state for relatively long periods. However, much of the ventilatory drive in these patients comes from hypoxic stimulation of the peripheral chemoreceptors discussed in Chapter 2. The arterial pH is nearly normal because of renal retention of bicarbonate (compensated respiratory acidosis), and the pH of the cerebrospinal fluid (CSF) is also normal (or nearly so) because of a compensatory increase in bicarbonate there. Thus despite an increased arterial P_{CO_2}, the main ventilatory drive comes from the hypoxemia.

If such a patient develops a relatively mild intercurrent respiratory infection that worsens the hypoxemia, and is therefore treated with a high inspired oxygen concentration, a potentially dangerous situation can rapidly develop. The hypoxic ventilatory drive may be abolished while the work of breathing is further increased because of retained secretions or bronchospasm. As a result, the ventilation may become grossly depressed, and high levels of arterial P_{CO_2} may develop quickly. A secondary cause of CO_2 retention in these patients may be a release of hypoxic vasoconstriction in poorly ventilated areas of lung. This can lead to worsening of the ventilation-perfusion inequality.

These patients can present a therapeutic dilemma. On the one hand, it is clearly essential to give some O_2 to relieve the life-threatening hypoxemia. On the other hand, O_2 administration is likely to cause severe CO_2 retention and respiratory acidosis. The answer is to give a relatively low concentration (24 to 28% O_2) and monitor the arterial blood gases frequently.

CO_2 retention increases cerebral blood flow, causing headache, raised CSF pressure, and sometimes papilledema (swelling of the optic disc). In practice, the cerebral effects of hypercapnia overlap with the effects of hypoxemia.

The resulting abnormalities include restlessness, tremor, slurred speech, and fluctuations of mood.

Acidosis in Respiratory Failure

The CO_2 retention causes respiratory acidosis that may be severe, especially after the injudicious administration of oxygen. However, patients who gradually develop respiratory failure may retain considerable amounts of bicarbonate, thus keeping the fall of pH in check (see Fig. 2–4B).

Metabolic acidosis frequently coexists with respiratory acidosis and complicates the acid-base abnormality. As we have seen, this is caused by the liberation of lactic acid from hypoxic tissues.

Role of Diaphragm Fatigue

Fatigue of the diaphragm can contribute to the hypoventilation of respiratory failure. The diaphragm (see Fig. 1–2) consists of striated skeletal muscle controlled by automatic and voluntary neural pathways via the phrenic nerves. Although the diaphragm is predominantly composed of slow twitch oxidative fibers and fast twitch oxidative-glycolytic fibers, which are relatively resistant to fatigue, this can occur if the work of breathing is greatly increased over a prolonged period. Fatigue can be defined as a loss of contractile force after work. It can be measured from the transdiaphragmatic pressure resulting from a maximum contraction, indirectly from the muscle relaxation time, or the electromyogram. Some patients with severe COPD continually breathe close to the work level at which fatigue occurs, and an exacerbation of infection can push them into a fatigue state. This will then result in hypoventilation, CO_2 retention, and severe hypoxemia. Because CO_2 retention impairs diaphragm contractility and severe hypoxemia accelerates the onset of fatigue, a vicious circle develops.

The dangers of diaphragm fatigue can be limited by reducing the work of breathing by treating bronchospasm and controlling infection, and by giving oxygen judiciously to relieve the hypoxemia. The force of contraction can be improved by a training program, for example, by breathing through inspiratory resistances. In addition, the administration of methylxanthines improves diaphragm contractility, and because these drugs also relieve bronchoconstriction, they are useful.

Types of Respiratory Failure

Acute Overwhelming Lung Disease

Many acute lung diseases, if severe enough, can lead to respiratory failure. These include infections such as fulminating bacterial or viral pneumonia, vascular diseases such as pulmonary embolism, and exposure to inhaled toxic gases such as chlorine or nitrogen oxides. Respiratory failure supervenes as the primary disease progresses, and profound hypoxemia, with or without hypercapnia, develops. Treatment of the underlying disease (e.g., antibiotics for bacterial pneumonias) is necessary. This group of conditions merges into ARDS (see below).

Neuromuscular Disorders

Neuromuscular disorders can cause severe hypoventilation, leading to respiratory failure. FIGURE 9–4 shows that the possible causes include: 1) depression of the respiratory center by drugs (especially barbiturates and the morphine derivatives) or anesthesia, 2) diseases of the medulla, including encephalitis, trauma, hemorrhage, or neoplasm (rare), 3) abnormalities of the spinal conducting pathways, as following high cervical dislocation, 4) anterior horn cell diseases, such as poliomyelitis, 5) diseases of the nerves to the respiratory muscles, including the Guillain-Barré syndrome and diphtheria, 6) diseases of the myoneural junction such as myasthenia gravis and anticholinesterase

poisoning, 7) diseases of the respiratory muscles (e.g., progressive muscular dystrophy), 8) thoracic cage abnormalities, such as crushed chest, and 9) upper airway obstruction, such as tracheal compression by a thymoma. The essential feature of these conditions is hypoventilation, leading to CO_2 retention with moderate hypoxemia (Fig. 9–3). Respiratory acidosis occurs, and the magnitude of the fall in pH depends on the rapidity of the increase in P_{CO_2} and the extent of the renal compensation (see Fig. 2–4B).

Mechanical ventilation is often necessary in these conditions and occasionally, as in bulbar poliomyelitis, may be required for months or even years. The lung itself is often normal in these conditions.

Acute on Chronic Lung Disease

This is an important and common group that includes patients with chronic bronchitis and emphysema, asthma, and cystic fibrosis. Many patients with COPD have a gradual downhill course with increasingly severe hypoxemia and CO_2 retention over months or years. Such patients are usually capable of limited physical activity, although both the arterial P_{O_2} and P_{CO_2} may be in the region of 50 mm Hg. This situation is not conventionally referred to as respiratory failure.

However, if such a patient develops even a mild exacerbation of the chest infection, the condition often deteriorates rapidly with profound hypoxemia, CO_2 retention, and respiratory acidosis. The reserves of pulmonary function are minimal, and any increase in the work of breathing or worsening of ventilation-perfusion relationships as a result of retained secretions or

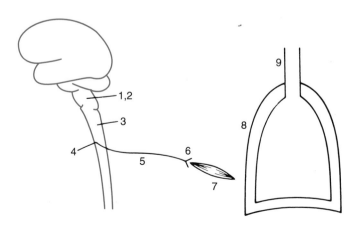

FIGURE 9–4. Causes of hypoventilation. (See text for details.)

bronchospasm, pushes the patient over the brink into frank respiratory failure.

The infection should be treated with antibiotics, bronchodilators may be indicated for bronchospasm, and diuretics and digitalis may be required if there is evidence of heart failure. Supplemental oxygen is often necessary to relieve severe hypoxemia. However, as discussed earlier in this chapter, these patients frequently lose their ventilatory drive and develop severe CO_2 retention and acidosis if too much oxygen is administered. For this reason, 24 to 28% oxygen should be given, and the arterial blood gases should be monitored frequently.

Adult Respiratory Distress Syndrome

This condition is also referred to as *acute respiratory failure*. The patient, Ivan, whose case was presented at the beginning of this chapter, is an example of someone with this condition. The condition is an end result of a variety of insults, including trauma to the lung or to the rest of the body (as in the case of Ivan), aspiration, sepsis (especially that caused by gram-negative organisms), and shock from any cause. Many other organs are also affected, and the condition can be regarded as multi-organ failure.

The early pathological changes in the lung include interstitial and alveolar edema. These progress to hemorrhage, cellular debris, and proteinaceous fluid in the alveoli, together with hyaline membranes, and there is patchy atelectasis (Fig. 9–2). Later, hyperplasia and organization occur. The damaged alveolar epithelium becomes lined with type II alveolar cells, and there is cellular infiltration of the alveolar walls. Sometimes interstitial fibrosis develops, although complete healing can occur.

The pathogenesis is unclear, and many factors probably play a role. The capillary endothelial and type I alveolar epithelial cells are damaged early, causing increased capillary permeability and flooding of the alveoli with proteinaceous fluid. Neutrophils accumulate partly as a result of complement or kinin activation. The activated neutrophils release mediators, including bradykinin, histamine, and platelet activating factor (PAF). In addition, toxic oxygen radicals are generated, together with cyclooxygenase products such as prostaglandins and thromboxane, and also lipoxygenase products such as leukotrienes (*see* Fig. 6–10). Platelets activated by PAF release proteases and kallikrein.

Pulmonary function is grossly impaired. The lung becomes very stiff, and unusually high pressures are required to ventilate it mechanically. The reduced compliance causes a marked fall in FRC. As would be expected from the histological appearance shown in Figure 9–2, there is severe ventilation-perfusion inequality, with a substantial fraction of the total blood flow going to unventilated alveoli. This shunt fraction may reach 50% or more. These patients need intubation and mechanical ventilation (as in the case of Ivan), and oxygen concentrations of 40 to 100% are sometimes necessary to maintain an arterial P_{O_2} above 60 mm Hg. The addition of positive end-expiratory pressure (PEEP) often results in substantial improvement in the arterial P_{O_2}, although high levels of lung inflation should be avoided if possible because they can damage the capillaries (see below).

Some of these patients have a low arterial P_{CO_2} even when severe hypoxemia develops (Fig. 9–3). The reason for the increased ventilation is not known, but possibly the interstitial edema stimulates intrapulmonary J or stretch receptors.

Infant Respiratory Distress Syndrome

This condition, which is also called *hyaline membrane disease of the newborn*, has several features in common with ARDS. Pathologically, the lung shows hemorrhagic edema, patchy atelectasis, and hyaline membranes caused by proteinaceous fluid and cellular debris within the alveoli (*see* Fig. 6–14). Physiologically, there is profound hypoxemia, with both ventilation-perfusion inequality and blood flow through unventilated lung. In addition, a right-to-left shunt via the patent foramen ovale may exaggerate hypoxemia. Mechanical ventilation with oxygen-enriched mixtures is often necessary, and the addition of PEEP or continuous positive airway pressure is frequently beneficial.

The chief cause of this condition is an absence of pulmonary surfactant (as discussed in Chapter 6), but other factors are probably also involved. The surfactant system of the lung matures relatively late in fetal life; therefore, infants born prematurely are particularly at risk. The ability of the infant to secrete surfactant can be estimated by measuring the lecithin/sphingomyelin ratio of amniotic fluid, and maturation of the surfactant-synthesizing system can be hastened by the administration of corticosteroids.

Treatment of the condition by instilling exogenous surfactant into the trachea is now effective.

☐ OXYGEN THERAPY

Oxygen administration has a critical role in the treatment of hypoxemia and especially in the management of respiratory failure. However, patients vary considerably in their response to oxygen, and there are several potential hazards associated with its use.

Response to Oxygen Administration

This depends on the mechanism of the hypoxemia. If this is caused by *hypoventilation*, small increases in the inspired O_2 concentration are very efficacious. This can be seen from the alveolar gas equation:

$$P_{A_{O_2}} = P_{I_{O_2}} - \frac{P_{A_{CO_2}}}{R} + F$$

where F is a small correction factor which can usually be ignored. The equation shows that if the alveolar P_{CO_2} and respiratory exchange ratio remain constant, and we neglect the correction factor, the alveolar P_{O_2} rises by 1 mm Hg for each mm Hg increase in inspired P_{O_2}. As an example, changing the inspired gas from air to only 30% O_2 will increase the alveolar P_{O_2} by approximately 60 mm Hg. The arterial P_{O_2} will rise by approximately the same amount.

If the hypoxemia is caused by *diffusion impairment*, O_2 administration is again very effective. The reason is that by raising the alveolar P_{O_2}, the driving pressure for O_2 across the blood-gas barrier is greatly increased (*see* Fig. 1–8). As a consequence, a modest rise in inspired oxygen concentration can often correct the hypoxemia.

If *ventilation-perfusion inequality* is the mechanism of the hypoxemia, O_2 administration is also usually very effective. If all the alveoli are ventilated, the alveolar P_{O_2} in them will eventually reach very high values as the nitrogen is washed out, and the arterial P_{O_2} will increase substantially. However, there are two cautions. First, if some regions of the lung are very poorly ventilated but perfused, it may take many minutes for the nitrogen to be washed out. Second, giving oxygen may result in the conversion of poorly ventilated areas into nonventilated areas, causing a shunt (see below). Nevertheless, O_2 therapy in

patients with ventilation-perfusion inequality is usually very effective in raising the arterial P_{O_2}.

Shunt is the only mechanism of hypoxemia in which arterial P_{O_2} responds much less to 100% O_2 breathing (*see* Fig. 7–6). The reason is that the blood that bypasses the ventilated alveoli is not exposed to the added oxygen, and it therefore continues to depress the arterial P_{O_2} (*see* Fig. 7–7). This means that giving 100% O_2 is a very sensitive way of detecting the presence of shunts.

However, it should be emphasized that useful gains in arterial P_{O_2} often follow the administration of 100% O_2 to patients with shunts. This is because of the additional dissolved oxygen, which can be appreciable at high alveolar P_{O_2} values. For example, increasing the alveolar P_{O_2} from 100 to 600 mm Hg raises the dissolved oxygen in the end-capillary blood from about 0.3 to 1.8 ml · dl^{-1}. This increase of 1.5 can be compared with the normal arterial-venous difference in O_2 concentration of approximately 5 ml · dl^{-1}.

FIGURE 9–5 shows typical increases in arterial P_{O_2} for various percentage shunts at different inspired O_2 concentrations. The graph is drawn for an O_2 uptake of 300 ml · min^{-1} and cardiac output of 6 l · min^{-1}, and variations in these and other values alter the positions of the lines.

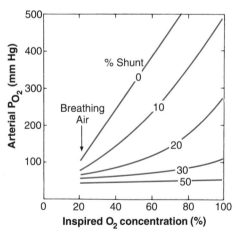

FIGURE 9–5. Response of the arterial P_{O_2} to increased inspired O_2 concentrations in a lung with various amounts of shunt. The P_{O_2} remains well below the normal level for 100% O_2 breathing. Nevertheless, useful gains in oxygenation occur even with severe degrees of shunting. (This theoretical diagram shows typical values only. Changes in cardiac output, oxygen uptake, etc. will affect the position of the lines.)

However, in this typical example, a patient with a shunt of 30% of the cardiac output who has an arterial P_{O_2} of 55 mm Hg during air breathing increases the P_{O_2} to 110 mm Hg when 100% O_2 is breathed. This increase corresponds to a rise in O_2 saturation and concentration of the arterial blood of 10% and 2.2 ml · dl^{-1}, respectively. In a patient with a severely hypoxic myocardium, such as George in Chapter 7, these values mean an important gain in O_2 delivery.

Other Factors in Oxygen Delivery

Although the arterial P_{O_2} is a convenient measurement of the degree of oxygenation of the blood, it is important to remember that other factors affect oxygen delivery to the tissues. These include the hemoglobin concentration, the position of the O_2 dissociation curve, the cardiac output, and the distribution of blood flow to the peripheral tissues.

Both a fall in hemoglobin concentration and cardiac output reduce the total amount of oxygen per unit time going to the tissues (*oxygen delivery* or *oxygen flux*). This can be expressed as the product of cardiac output and arterial O_2 concentration: $\dot{Q} \times Ca_{O_2}$.

Diffusion of O_2 from the peripheral capillaries to the mitochondria in the tissue cells depends on the capillary P_{O_2}. A useful index is the P_{O_2} of mixed venous blood, which is often taken as a measure of the average tissue P_{O_2}. A rearrangement of the Fick equation is as follows:

$$C\bar{v}_{O_2} = Ca_{O_2} - \frac{\dot{V}_{O_2}}{\dot{Q}}$$

This equation shows that the O_2 concentration (and therefore the P_{O_2}) of mixed venous blood will fall if either the arterial O_2 concentration or the cardiac output is reduced (O_2 consumption assumed constant).

The relationship between O_2 concentration and P_{O_2} in the mixed venous blood depends on the position of the O_2 dissociation curve (*see* Fig. 1–15). If the curve is shifted to the right by an increase in temperature, as in fever, or an increase in 2,3-DPG concentration, as frequently occurs in chronic hypoxemia, the P_{O_2} for a given O_2 concentration is high, thus favoring diffusion of O_2 to the mitochondria. By contrast, if the P_{CO_2} is low and the pH is high, as in respiratory alkalosis, or if the 2,3-DPG concentration is low because of transfusion of large amounts of stored blood in which the

2,3-DPG has been depleted, the resulting left-shifted curve interferes with O_2 unloading to the tissues.

Methods of Oxygen Administration

Nasal cannulas consist of two prongs that are inserted just inside the anterior nares and are supported on a light frame. Oxygen is supplied at rates of 1 to 4 l · min^{-1}, resulting in inspired O_2 concentrations of approximately 25 to 30%. The higher the patient's inspiratory flow rate, the lower the resulting concentration because of dilution with the inspired air. The O_2 should be humidified to prevent crusting of secretions. Cannulas are convenient because the patient does not have the discomfort of a mask and cannulas do not interfere with talking and eating. They can be worn continuously for long periods.

Masks come in several designs. Simple plastic masks that fit over the nose and mouth allow inspired O_2 concentrations of up to 60% when supplied with flow rates of 6 l · min^{-1}. However, some patients do not tolerate masks well.

A useful mask for delivering controlled O_2 concentrations is based on the Venturi principle. As the O_2 enters the mask through a narrow jet, it entrains a constant flow of air. With an oxygen flow of 4 l · min^{-1}, a total flow (O_2 plus air) of approximately 40 l · min^{-1} is delivered to the patient. Masks are available to give inspired O_2 concentrations of 24%, 28%, or 35% with a high degree of reliability and are particularly useful for treating patients who are liable to develop CO_2 retention if a higher concentration of O_2 is given.

Transtracheal oxygen can be delivered via a microcatheter inserted through the anterior tracheal wall with the tip lying just above the carina. This is an efficient way of delivering O_2 in patients who are receiving long-term oxygen therapy (see below).

Mechanical ventilators, when used in conjunction with an endotracheal tube, allow complete control over the composition of the inspired gas. The potentially high concentrations raise the dangers of O_2 toxicity (see below). In general, the lowest inspired O_2 concentration that provides an acceptable arterial P_{O_2} should be used. This level is difficult to define, but in patients with ARDS who are being mechanically ventilated with high O_2 concentrations, 60 mm Hg is often used.

Hyperbaric oxygen. If 100% O_2 is administered at a pressure of 3 atmospheres, the inspired P_{O_2} is over 2000 mm Hg. Under these conditions, a substantial increase in the arterial O_2 concentration can occur, chiefly as a result of the additional dissolved O_2. For example, if the arterial P_{O_2} is 2000 mm Hg, the O_2 in solution is approximately $6 \ ml \cdot dl^{-1}$ of blood. Theoretically, this is enough to provide the entire arterial-venous O_2 difference of $5 \ ml \cdot dl^{-1}$, so that the hemoglobin of the mixed venous blood could remain fully saturated.

Hyperbaric O_2 therapy has limited uses and is rarely indicated in the treatment of respiratory failure. However, it has been used in the treatment of severe carbon monoxide poisoning, in which most of the hemoglobin is unavailable to carry O_2, and therefore the dissolved O_2 is critically important. In addition, the high P_{O_2} accelerates the dissociation of carbon monoxide from hemoglobin. A severe anemic crisis is sometimes treated in the same way. Hyperbaric O_2 is also used in the treatment of gas gangrene infections and as an adjunct to radiotherapy, in which the higher tissue P_{O_2} increases the radio-sensitivity of relatively avascular tumors. The high pressure chamber is also valuable for managing decompression sickness after diving.

The use of hyperbaric O_2 requires a special facility with trained personnel. In practice, the chamber is filled with air and O_2 is given by a special mask to ensure that the patient receives pure O_2. This procedure also reduces fire hazard.

Domiciliary and portable oxygen are now frequently used by patients with severe COPD. These patients may be virtually confined to bed or a chair unless they breathe supplementary oxygen. Portable oxygen sets can be used for shopping and other outside activities.

Administration of a low flow of oxygen given continuously over several months can reduce the amount of pulmonary hypertension and improve the prognosis of some patients with advanced COPD. Although such therapy is expensive, improvements in technology, for example O_2 concentrators that remove O_2 from the air, have made this feasible.

Hazards of Oxygen Therapy

Carbon Dioxide Retention

As discussed earlier, patients with severe COPD who are given high concentrations of O_2 to breathe may develop dangerous CO_2 retention.

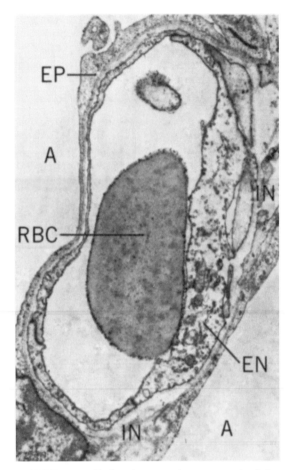

FIGURE 9–6. Early changes in oxygen toxicity. This electron micrograph from a monkey exposed to 100% O_2 for 2 days shows swelling of the capillary endothelial cells. Later changes include loss of alveolar epithelium and subsequent interstitial fibrosis. *A*, alveolus; *EN*, endothelium; *EP*, epithelium; *IN*, interstitium; *RBC*, red blood cell.

Oxygen should be given at relatively low concentrations, for example 24% via a Venturi mask, and the blood gases should be monitored.

Oxygen Toxicity

High concentrations of O_2 administered over long periods can damage the lung. If guinea pigs are placed in 100% O_2 at atmospheric pressure for 48 hours, they develop pulmonary edema. **FIGURE 9–6** shows an electron micrograph from a monkey exposed to 100% O_2 for 2 days (compare with Fig. 1–7). Note the swollen capillary endothelium, which is where some of the earliest changes are seen. Alterations also occur in the endothelial intercellular junctions.

The alveolar epithelium may become completely denuded and replaced by rows of type II epithelial cells. There is an increased capillary permeability that leads to interstitial and alveolar edema. Later, organization occurs with interstitial fibrosis.

In humans, the pulmonary effects of high O_2 concentrations are more difficult to document, but normal subjects report substernal discomfort after breathing 100% O_2 for 24 hours. Patients who have been mechanically ventilated with 100% O_2 for 36 hours have shown a progressive fall in arterial P_{O_2}, compared with a control group who were ventilated with air. A reasonable attitude is to assume that concentrations of 50% O_2 or higher for more than 2 days may produce toxic changes.

In practice, such high levels of O_2 over such a long period can only be achieved in patients who are intubated and mechanically ventilated. It is important to avoid oxygen toxicity because the only way to relieve the resultant hypoxemia is by raising the inspired O_2, thus creating a vicious circle.

Atelectasis

Following airway occlusion. Absorption atelectasis is an important hazard of breathing 100% O_2.

Suppose that an airway is obstructed by mucus (**FIGURE 9–7A**). The total pressure in the trapped gas is close to 760 mm Hg (it may be a few mm Hg less as it is absorbed because of elastic forces in the lung), but the sum of the partial pressures in the venous blood is far less than 760 mm Hg. This is because the P_{O_2} of the mixed venous blood remains relatively low, even when O_2 is breathed. In fact, the Fick equation shows that the rise in O_2 *concentration* of arterial and venous blood when O_2 is breathed will be the same if cardiac output and oxygen uptake remain unchanged. However, because of the shape of the O_2 dissociation curve (*see* Fig. 1–14), the increase in venous P_{O_2} is only about 10 to 15 mm Hg, in contrast to the very large increase in arterial P_{O_2}. Since the sum of the partial pressures in the alveolar gas greatly exceeds that in venous blood, gas diffuses into the blood, and rapid collapse of the alveoli occurs. Reopening such an atelectatic area may be difficult because of surface tension effects in such small units.

Absorption atelectasis also occurs in a blocked region of lung, even when air is breathed, although here the process is slower. Figure 9–7B shows that, again, the sum of the partial pressures in venous blood is less than 760 mm Hg. This is because the fall in P_{O_2} from arterial to

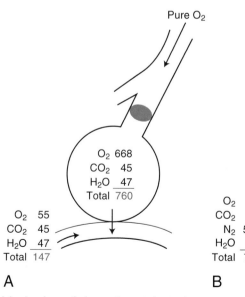 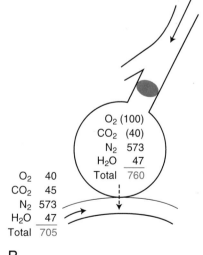

A   B

FIGURE 9–7. Mechanism of absorption atelectasis beyond blocked airways. **A.** Partial pressures when 100% O_2 is inspired. **B.** Partial pressures when air is breathed. In both cases, the sum of the partial pressures of the gases in the mixed venous blood is less than that in the alveoli. In **B,** the P_{O_2} and P_{CO_2} are shown in parentheses because these values change with time. However, the total alveolar pressure remains within a few mm Hg of 760.

venous blood is much greater than the rise in P_{CO_2} (this is a reflection of the steeper slope of the CO_2 dissociation curve [see Fig. 1–17], compared with the O_2 dissociation curve [see Fig. 1–14]). Since the total gas pressure in the alveoli is nearly 760 mm Hg, absorption is inevitable.

The changes in the alveolar partial pressures during absorption are somewhat complicated, but it can be shown that the rate of collapse is limited by the rate of absorption of nitrogen. Since this gas has a low solubility, its presence acts as a "splint" that, as it were, supports the alveoli and delays collapse. Even relatively small concentrations of nitrogen in alveolar gas have a useful splinting effect. Nevertheless, postoperative atelectasis is a common problem in patients who are treated with high O_2 mixtures. Collapse is particularly likely to occur at the bottom of the lung, where the parenchyma is least well expanded (see Fig. 3–11) or the airways are actually closed (see Fig. 3–12). Also, retained secretions tend to collect at the lung base because they drain there. This same basic mechanism of absorption is responsible for the gradual disappearance of pneumothorax or a gas pocket inadvertently introduced under the skin.

Instability of units with low ventilation-perfusion ratios. Lung units with low ventilation-perfusion ratios may become unstable and collapse when high O_2 mixtures are inhaled. An example is given in **FIGURE 9–8**, which shows the distribution of ventilation-perfusion ratios in a patient during air breathing and again after 30 minutes of breathing 100% O_2. This patient had acute respiratory failure following an automobile accident, as was the case with Ivan. During air breathing, there were appreciable amounts of blood flow to lung units with ventilation-perfusion ratios between 0.01 and 0.1. There was also an 8% shunt, that is, blood flow to completely unventilated lung units. After O_2 administration, the blood flow to the low ventilation-perfusion ratio units was not seen, but the shunt had increased from 8 to 16%. The most likely explanation of these changes is that the poorly ventilated regions became unventilated.

FIGURE 9–9 shows the mechanism. Here we see four hypothetical lung units, all with low inspired ventilation-perfusion ratios ($\dot{V}_{AI}/\dot{Q}$) during 80% O_2 breathing. In A, the inspired (alveolar) ventilation is 49.4 units, but the expired ventilation is only 2.5 units (the actual values depend on the blood flow). The reason why so little gas is exhaled is that so much is taken up by the blood. In B, where the inspired ventilation is slightly reduced to 44 units (same blood flow as before), there is no expired ventilation at all because all the gas that is inspired is absorbed by the blood. Such a unit is said to have a "critical" ventilation-perfusion ratio. In C and D, the inspired ventilation has been further reduced with the result that it is now less than the volume of gas entering the blood. This is an unstable situation. Under these circumstances, either gas is inspired from neigh-

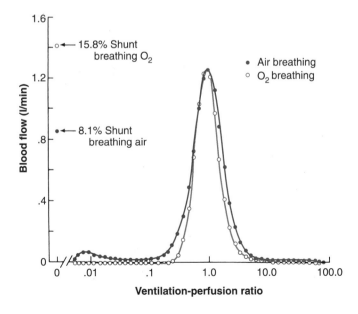

FIGURE 9–8. Conversion of low ventilation-perfusion ratio units to shunt during O_2 breathing. This patient had acute respiratory failure following an automobile accident. During air breathing, there was appreciable blood flow to units with low ventilation-perfusion ratios. After 30 minutes of breathing 100% O_2, blood flow to these units was not seen, but the shunt doubled.

Inspired $O_2 = 80\%$

$\dot{V}_{AI}/\dot{Q}$ 0.0494   0.0440   0.0373   0.0373

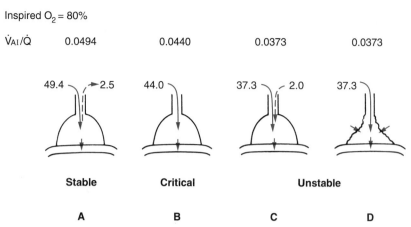

Stable	Critical	Unstable
A	B	C	D

FIGURE 9–9. Mechanism of the collapse of lung units with low inspired ventilation-perfusion ratios ($\dot{V}_{AI}/\dot{Q}$) when high O_2 mixtures are inhaled. **A.** The expired ventilation is very small because so much of the inspired gas is taken up by the blood. **C** and **D.** More gas is removed from the lung unit than is inspired, leading to an unstable condition.

boring units during the expiratory phase of respiration, as in C, or the unit gradually collapses, as in D. The latter fate is particularly likely if the unit is poorly ventilated because of intermittent airway closure. This is probably common in the dependent regions of the lung in many patients with acute respiratory failure, such as that caused by ARDS, because of the greatly reduced FRC. The likelihood of atelectasis increases rapidly as the inspired O_2 concentration approaches 100%.

The development of shunts during O_2 breathing is an additional reason why high concentrations of O_2 should be avoided if possible in the treatment of patients with respiratory failure. Also, if a shunt is measured during 100% O_2 breathing (*see* Fig. 7–7) in these patients, it may substantially overestimate the shunt that is present during air breathing.

Retrolental Fibroplasia

If newborn infants with the infant respiratory distress syndrome are treated with high concentrations of O_2, they may develop fibrosis behind the lens of the eye, leading to blindness. To avoid this, the arterial P_{O_2} should be kept below 140 mm Hg.

☐ MECHANICAL VENTILATION

We saw that it was necessary to use mechanical ventilation in the management of Ivan because his acute respiratory failure had caused such severe impairment of gas exchange that it was impossible to maintain viable levels of arterial P_{O_2} and P_{CO_2} without this intervention. Mechanical ventilation is frequently used in the intensive care environment. This is a complex and technical subject, and the present discussion is limited to the physiological principles of its use, benefits, and hazards.

Intubation and Tracheostomy

Most ventilators require a port for connection to the lung airway. An exception is the tank type of ventilator (see below), which is now rarely used. The connection is made by means of an endotracheal (or sometimes tracheostomy) tube. These are provided with an inflatable cuff at the end to give an airtight seal. Endotracheal tubes are usually inserted via the nose.

These tubes have other functions in addition to providing a connection for ventilators. They facilitate the removal of retained secretions by suction catheter, a serious problem in many patients with respiratory failure. These secretions are particularly troublesome in patients who are semiconscious, or who have a suppressed cough reflex, or when the secretions are particularly copious or viscid. In addition, a tracheostomy may be necessary to bypass upper airway obstruction caused, for example, by allergic edema or a laryngeal tumor. The tube may also prevent the aspiration of blood or vomitus from the pharynx into the lung.

The decision to intubate and ventilate a patient is a major one because the intervention requires a large investment of personnel and equipment, with many potential hazards. However, patients are frequently intubated too late in the course of respiratory failure. The precise timing depends on a number of factors including the nature of the underlying disease process, the rapidity of the progress of hypoxemia and hypercapnia, and the age and general condition of the patient.

Several complications are associated with the use of endotracheal and tracheostomy tubes. Ulceration of the larynx or trachea is sometimes seen. This complication is particularly likely if the inflated cuff exerts undue pressure on the mucosa. The subsequent scarring can result in tracheal stenosis. The use of large-volume, low-pressure cuffs has reduced the incidence of this problem. Care must be taken with the placement of an endotracheal tube. Occasionally the distal end of the tube is inadvertently placed in the right main bronchus, leading to atelectasis of the left lung.

Types of Ventilators

Constant-Volume Ventilators

These ventilators deliver a preset volume of gas to the patient, usually by means of a motor-driven piston in a cylinder (FIGURE 9–10). The stroke and frequency of the pump can be adjusted to give the required ventilation, and the ratio of inspiratory to expiratory time can also be controlled. Oxygen can be added to the inspired gas as required, and a humidifier is included in the circuit. Constant-volume ventilators are robust, dependable machines that are suitable for long-term ventilation. They are used extensively in anesthesia.

Constant-Pressure Ventilators

These ventilators deliver gas at a preset pressure. They do not require electrical power but instead work from a source of compressed gas. They can include a valve that allows inspiration to be triggered by a patient's inspiratory effort. Constant-pressure ventilators are small, relatively inexpensive machines. A potential disadvantage is that the volume of gas they deliver is altered by changes in the compliance of the lung or chest wall.

Tank Ventilators

Although these are uncommon now, they were extensively used to ventilate patients with bulbar poliomyelitis, and they are still occasionally useful for patients with chronic neuromuscular disease. In contrast to the positive-pressure ventilators considered so far, they work by delivering negative pressure (less than atmospheric) to the outside of the chest and rest of

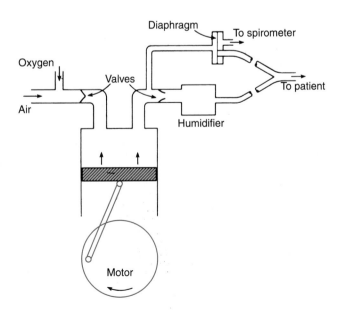

FIGURE 9–10. Diagram of a constant-volume ventilator. In practice, the stroke volume and frequency of the pump can be regulated. During the expiratory phase the piston descends, and the diaphragm is deflected to the left by the reduced pressure in the cylinder, allowing the patient to exhale through the spirometer.

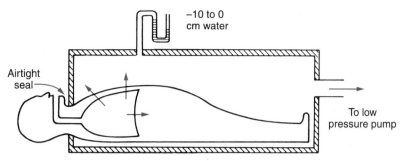

FIGURE 9–11. Tank respirator (schematic). The rigid box is connected to a large-volume, low-pressure pump which swings the pressure from about 0 to –10 cm H_2O.

the body, excluding the head (**FIGURE 9–11**). The ventilator consists of a rigid box ("iron lung") connected to a large-volume, low-pressure pump that controls the respiratory cycle. The box is often hinged along the middle so that it can be opened to allow nursing care. A modification of the tank ventilator is the cuirass which fits over the thorax and abdomen and also generates negative pressure. It is usually reserved for patients who have partially recovered from neuromuscular respiratory failure.

Patterns of Ventilation

Positive End-Expiratory Pressure

In many patients with acute respiratory failure, considerable improvement in the arterial P_{O_2} can be obtained by maintaining a small positive airway pressure at the end of expiration. Values as low as 5 cm H_2O are often beneficial, but pressures as high as 20 cm H_2O or more are sometimes necessary, although high pressures should be avoided if possible (see below). Special valves are available to provide the pressure. A secondary gain from PEEP is that it may allow the inspired O_2 concentration to be decreased, thus lessening the risk of O_2 toxicity.

Several mechanisms are responsible for the increase in arterial P_{O_2} when PEEP is applied. The positive pressure increases the FRC, which is typically small in these patients because of the increased elastic recoil of the lung. The low lung volume causes airway closure and intermittent ventilation (or none at all) of some areas, especially in the dependent regions, and absorption atelectasis ensues (Fig. 9–9). PEEP tends to reverse these changes. Patients with edema in their airways also benefit, probably because the fluid is moved into small peripheral airways,

allowing some regions of the lung to be reventilated.

FIGURE 9–12 shows the effects of PEEP in a patient with ARDS. The level of PEEP was progressively increased from 0 to 16 cm H_2O, and this resulted in the shunt falling from 43.8 to 14.2% of the total pulmonary blood flow. A small amount of blood flow to very poorly ventilated alveoli remained. In this patient, the arterial P_{O_2} with zero PEEP (sometimes called ZEEP) was only 73 mm Hg when the patient was ventilated with 80% O_2.

Figure 9–12 also shows that the addition of PEEP increased the dead space from 36.3 to 49.8% of the tidal volume. This can be explained partly by compression of the capillaries by the increased alveolar pressure and is the same basic mechanism that is responsible for the development of zone I in the distribution of blood flow in the lung, as discussed in connection with Figure 6–7. **FIGURE 9–13** shows the collapse of capillaries in the alveolar wall when alveolar pressure is raised above capillary pressure and should be contrasted with the normal appearance shown in Figure 1–12. These lung units are useless for gas exchange and this is an example of alveolar dead space. In addition, PEEP results in an increase in the volume of the conducting airways (anatomic dead space) because of the increase in volume of the lung and consequent increased radial traction on the airways.

A related consequence of PEEP is its tendency to reduce cardiac output by impeding venous return to the thorax. This is particularly likely to occur if the circulating blood volume has been depleted by hemorrhage or shock. Therefore, the value of PEEP should not be gauged only by its effect on the arterial P_{O_2}, but also in terms of the total amount of oxygen delivered to the tissues (cardiac output × arterial

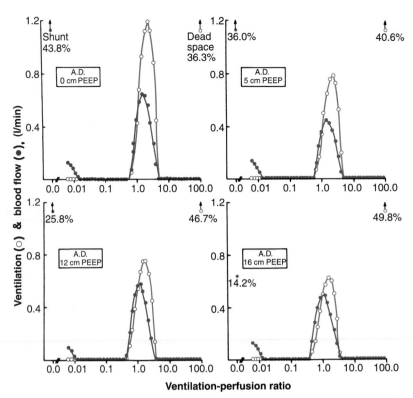

FIGURE 9–12. Reduction of shunt and increase of dead space caused by increasing levels of PEEP in a patient with ARDS. As the PEEP was progressively increased from 0 to 16 cm H₂O, the shunt decreased from 43.8 to 14.2% of the total blood flow, and the dead space increased from 36.3 to 49.8% of the tidal volume.

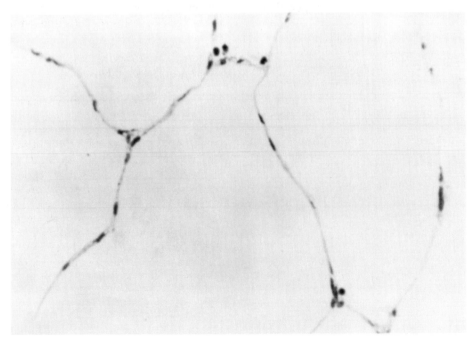

FIGURE 9–13. Effect of raising airway pressure on the histological appearance of pulmonary capillaries. Compare with the normal appearance as shown in Figure 1–12. When alveolar pressure was raised above capillary pressure, the capillaries collapsed and few red blood cells remained in the alveolar walls.

O_2 concentration). Because the P_{O_2} of mixed venous blood reflects the oxygen delivery to the tissues (if O_2 uptake is constant), some physicians use the P_{O_2} of mixed venous blood as a guide to the optimal level of PEEP.

However, in some extremely ill patients, this can be a misleading measurement. Under some conditions, the application of PEEP causes a reduction in the patient's overall O_2 consumption. The reason is that the perfusion of some tissues in extremely ill patients is so marginal that if the blood flow is further decreased, they are unable to take up oxygen.

It is now well-established that high levels of PEEP can damage pulmonary capillaries, leading to pulmonary edema. The mechanism is that the very high levels of alveolar distension (at least in some regions of the lung) cause such high mechanical tension in the alveolar walls that the very thin blood-gas barrier is damaged (stress failure). In general, therefore, very high levels of PEEP should be avoided, and the lowest pressure consistent with an acceptable level of arterial P_{O_2} should be used. Sometimes reducing the level of PEEP results in CO_2 retention, but recent evidence suggests that this is less deleterious in some patients than the capillary damage that otherwise occurs. If the P_{CO_2} is allowed to rise, the situation is sometimes referred to as permissive hypercapnia.

Occasionally, the addition of too much PEEP reduces rather than increases the arterial P_{O_2}. Possible mechanisms include the fall in cardiac output which reduces the P_{O_2} of mixed venous blood and therefore the arterial P_{O_2}, reduced ventilation of well-perfused regions of lung, and diversion of blood flow away from ventilated to unventilated regions. However, these possible disadvantages should not obscure the fact that PEEP is a very important treatment option in the management of patients with severe respiratory failure.

Other Patterns of Ventilation

Several special patterns of mechanical ventilation are used but the details need not concern us.

Intermittent positive pressure ventilation (IPPV) is the common pattern, in which the lung is expanded by the application of positive pressure to the airway and allowed to deflate passively to FRC. In some patients with airway obstruction, there is an advantage in prolonging the expiratory time so that all regions of the lung have time to empty. This can be done by reducing the respiratory frequency and increasing the expiratory versus inspiratory time. *Continuous positive airway pressure* (CPAP) is sometimes used when patients are being weaned from a ventilator and are able to breathe spontaneously. These patients may benefit from a small positive pressure applied continuously to the airway. The result is an improvement in oxygenation. CPAP is also used in treating sleep-disordered breathing caused by upper airway obstruction.

Intermittent mandatory ventilation (IMV) is a modification of IPPV in which a large tidal volume is given at relatively infrequent intervals to an intubated patient who is breathing spontaneously. It is often combined with PEEP or CPAP. *High frequency ventilation* is a specialized form of mechanical ventilation in which very high frequency (approximately 20 cycles $\cdot$ sec^{-1}) positive pressure ventilation is applied with very small stroke volumes (50 to 100 ml). As a result, the lung is vibrated rather than expanded in the conventional way, and the transport of gas occurs by a combination of diffusion and convection.

Miscellaneous Hazards

Mechanical problems are a constant hazard. They include power failure, broken connections, and kinking of tubes. *Pneumothorax* can occur, especially if high levels of PEEP or unusually large tidal volumes are used. *Interstitial emphysema* may occur if the lung is overdistended and air escapes from ruptured alveoli into the perivascular and peribronchial interstitium (*see* Figs. 7–2 and 7–3). The air may enter the mediastinum and the subcutaneous tissues of the neck. *Pulmonary infection* can occur, and *cardiac arrhythmias* may be caused by rapid swings in pH and also hypoxemia.

Questions

For each question, choose the one best answer.
(For answers, see p. 150.)

1. Severe hypoxemia, as in acute respiratory failure, can cause all of the following EXCEPT:
   A. Tachycardia
   B. Nystagmus
   C. Lactic acidemia
   D. Proteinuria
   E. Mental clouding

2. Severe carbon dioxide retention can cause all of the following EXCEPT:
   A. Mental clouding
   B. Acidosis
   C. Reduced cerebral blood flow
   D. Renal retention of bicarbonate
   E. Raised CSF pressure

3. All of the following statements about the diaphragm are true EXCEPT:
   A. It is composed of striated skeletal muscle.
   B. It is under both automatic and voluntary control.
   C. Nerve supply is via cervical segments 3, 4, and 5.
   D. Fatigue results in a reduced maximal transdiaphragmatic pressure.
   E. Diaphragm function cannot be improved by a training program.

4. Features of ARDS typically include the following EXCEPT:
   A. Severe hypoxemia
   B. Ventilation-perfusion inequality without a shunt
   C. Reduced lung compliance
   D. Reduced FRC
   E. Obvious opacification of the chest radiograph

5. Features of infant respiratory distress syndrome typically include all of the following EXCEPT:
   A. Patchy hemorrhagic edema and atelectasis
   B. Production of an abnormal form of pulmonary surfactant

C. Severe hypoxemia
D. Large shunt
E. Increased risk in premature infants

6. A patient with COPD developed an acute exacerbation of his bronchitis and was admitted to the hospital. When he was given 100% O_2, his arterial Pco_2 increased from 45 to 60 mm Hg. All of the following statements are true EXCEPT:
   A. The exacerbation of his infection increased ventilation-perfusion inequality.
   B. Administration of oxygen released hypoxic vasoconstriction in some poorly ventilated areas of lung.
   C. Administration of oxygen depressed ventilation.
   D. The patient should be intubated immediately.
   E. The patient should be given a lower concentration of oxygen, and the blood gases should be monitored.

7. A young man who was previously well was admitted to the emergency department with barbiturate poisoning that caused severe hypoventilation. When he was given 50% O_2 to breathe, there was no change in his arterial Pco_2. Approximately how much would his arterial Po_2 (mm Hg) be expected to rise?
   A. 25
   B. 50
   C. 75
   D. 100
   E. 200

8. Hyperbaric oxygen therapy can be useful in all of the following conditions EXCEPT:
   A. Severe carbon monoxide poisoning
   B. Gas gangrene infections

C. Radiotherapy of some malignant tumors
D. Spontaneous pneumothorax
E. An acute anemic crisis

9. **A patient with ARDS is treated by mechanical ventilation. Adding 15 cm H_2O of positive end-expiratory pressure** (**PEEP**) **typically has the following effects EXCEPT:**
   A. Increased FRC
   B. Reduced shunt
   C. Increased alveolar edema
   D. Increased physiological dead space
   E. Reduced venous return to the thorax

Appendix A

Symbols, Units, Equations, and Normal Values

Symbols

Primary Symbols

C   Concentration of gas in blood
F   Fractional concentration in dry gas
P   Pressure or partial pressure
Q   Volume of blood
$\dot{Q}$ Volume of blood per unit time
R   Respiratory exchange ratio
S   Saturation of hemoglobin with O_2
V   Volume of gas
$\dot{V}$ Volume of gas per unit time

Secondary Symbols for Gas Phase

A   Alveolar
B   Barometric
D   Dead space
E   Expired
I   Inspired
L   Lung
T   Tidal

Secondary Symbols for Blood Phase

a   arterial
c   capillary
c´   end-capillary
i   ideal
v   venous
$\bar{v}$ mixed venous

Examples

O_2 concentration in arterial blood, Ca_{O_2}
Fractional concentration of N_2 in expired gas, $F_{E_{N_2}}$
Partial pressure of O_2 in mixed venous blood, $P\bar{v}_{O_2}$

Units

Traditional metric units have been used in this book. Pressures are given in mm Hg; the torr is an almost identical unit.

In Europe, SI (Système International) units are commonly used. Most of these are familiar, but the kilopascal, the unit of pressure, is confusing at first. One kilopascal = 7.5 mm Hg (approximately).

Equations

Gas Laws

General gas law:

$$PV = RT$$

where T is temperature and R is a constant. This equation is used to correct gas volumes for changes of water vapor pressure and temperature. For example, ventilation is conventionally reported at BTPS, that is, body temperature (37°C), ambient pressure, and saturated with water vapor because it then corresponds to the volume changes of the lung. By contrast, gas volumes in blood are expressed as STPD, that is, standard temperature (0°C or 273°K) and pressure (760 mm Hg) and dry as is usual in chemistry. To convert a gas volume at BTPS to one at STPD, multiply by:

$$\frac{273}{310} \times \frac{P_B - 47}{760}$$

where 47 mm Hg is the water vapor pressure at 37°C.
Boyle's law

$$P_1V_1 = P_2V_2 \quad \text{(temperature constant)}$$

and *Charles' law*

$$\frac{V_1}{V_2} = \frac{T_1}{T_2} \quad \text{(pressure constant)}$$

are special cases of the general gas law.
Avogadro's law states that equal volumes of different gases at the same temperature and pressure contain the same number of molecules. A gram molecule, for example, 32 gm of O_2, occupies 22.4 liters at STPD.
Dalton's law states that the partial pressure of a gas (x) in a gas mixture is the pressure that this gas would exert if it occupied the total volume of the mixture in the absence of the other components.
Thus, $P_x = P \cdot F_x$, where P is the total dry gas pressure, since F_x refers to dry gas. In gas with a water vapor pressure of 47 mm Hg,

$$P_x = (P_B - 47) \cdot F_x$$

Also, in the alveoli, $P_{O_2} + P_{CO_2} + P_{N_2} + P_{H_2O} = P_B$.
The *partial pressure of a gas in solution* is its partial pressure in a gas mixture that is in equilibrium with the solution.
Henry's law states that the concentration of gas dissolved in a liquid is proportional to its partial pressure. Thus, $C_x = K \cdot P_x$.

Ventilation

$$V_T = V_D + V_A$$

where V_A here refers to the volume of alveolar gas in the tidal volume:

$$\dot{V}_A = \dot{V}_E - \dot{V}_D$$

$$\dot{V}_{CO_2} = \dot{V}_A \cdot F_{ACO_2} \quad \text{(both measured at BTPS)}$$

$$\dot{V}_A = \frac{\dot{V}_{CO_2}}{P_{ACO_2}} \times K \quad \text{(alveolar ventilation equation)}$$

If $\dot{V}_A$ is BTPS and $\dot{V}_{CO_2}$ is STPD, $K = 0.863$. In normal subjects P_{ACO_2} is nearly identical to P_{ACO_2}.

Bohr equation:

$$\frac{V_D}{V_T} = \frac{P_{ACO_2} - P_{ECO_2}}{P_{ACO_2}}$$

Or, using arterial P_{CO_2}:

$$\frac{V_D}{V_T} = \frac{P_{aCO_2} - P_{ECO_2}}{P_{aCO_2}}$$

This gives *physiologic dead space*.

Diffusion

In the *gas phase*, *Graham's law* states that the rate of diffusion of a gas is inversely proportional to the square root of its molecular weight.

In *liquid or a tissue slice*, *Fick's law** states that the volume of gas per unit time that diffuses across a tissue sheet is given by:

$$\dot{V}_{gas} = \frac{A}{T} \cdot D \cdot (P_1 - P_2)$$

where A and T are the area and thickness of the sheet, P_1 and P_2 are the partial pressure of the gas on the two sides, and D is a diffusion constant, sometimes called the permeability coefficient of the tissue for that gas.

This *diffusion constant* is related to the solubility (Sol) and the molecular weight (MW) of the gas:

$$D \, \alpha \, \frac{Sol}{\sqrt{MW}}$$

When the diffusing capacity of the lung (D_L) is measured with carbon monoxide and the capillary P_{CO} is taken as zero:

$$D_L = \frac{\dot{V}_{CO}}{P_{ACO}}$$

D_L is made up of two components. One is the diffusing capacity of the alveolar membrane (D_M), and the other depends on the volume of capillary blood (V_c) and the rate of reaction of CO with hemoglobin θ:

$$\frac{1}{D_L} = \frac{1}{D_M} + \frac{1}{\theta \cdot V_c}$$

Blood Flow

Fick principle:

$$\dot{Q} = \frac{\dot{V}_{O_2}}{Ca_{O_2} - C\bar{v}_{O_2}}$$

Pulmonary vascular resistance:

$$PVR = \frac{P_{art} - P_{ven}}{\dot{Q}}$$

where P_{art} and P_{ven} are the mean pulmonary arterial and venous pressures, respectively.

Starling's law of fluid exchange across the capillaries:

$$\text{Net flow out} = K[(P_c - P_i) - \sigma(\pi_c - \pi_i)]$$

where i refers to the interstitial fluid around the capillary, π to the colloid osmotic pressure, σ is the reflection coefficient, and K is the filtration coefficient.

Ventilation-Perfusion Relationships

Alveolar gas equation:

$$P_{AO_2} = P_{IO_2} - \frac{P_{ACO_2}}{R} + \left[P_{ACO_2} \cdot F_{IO_2} \cdot \frac{1-R}{R} \right]$$

This is only valid if there is no CO_2 in inspired gas. The term in square brackets is a relatively small correction factor when air is breathed (2 mm Hg when $P_{CO_2} = 40$, $F_{IO_2} = 0.21$, and $R = 0.8$). Thus, a useful approximation is:

$$P_{AO_2} = P_{IO_2} - \frac{P_{ACO_2}}{R}$$

Respiratory exchange ratio: If no CO_2 is present in the inspired gas,

$$R = \frac{\dot{V}_{CO_2}}{\dot{V}_{O_2}} = \frac{P_{ECO_2}(1 - F_{IO_2})}{P_{IO_2} - P_{EO_2} - (P_{ECO_2} \cdot F_{IO_2})}$$

Venous to arterial shunt:

$$\frac{\dot{Q}_S}{\dot{Q}_T} = \frac{Cc'_{O_2} - Ca_{O_2}}{Cc'_{O_2} - C\bar{v}_{O_2}}$$

where c′ means end-capillary.

Ventilation-perfusion ratio equation:

$$\frac{\dot{V}_A}{\dot{Q}} = \frac{8.63R(Ca_{O_2} - C\bar{v}_{O_2})}{P_{ACO_2}}$$

where blood gas concentrations are in $ml \cdot dl^{-1}$.

---

* Fick's law was originally expressed in terms of concentrations, but partial pressures are more convenient for us.

Physiologic shunt:

$$\frac{\dot{Q}_{PS}}{\dot{Q}_T} = \frac{Ci_{O_2} - Ca_{O_2}}{Ci_{O_2} - C\overline{v}_{O_2}}$$

Alveolar dead space:

$$\frac{V_D}{V_T} = \frac{Pi_{CO_2} - P_{A_{CO_2}}}{Pi_{CO_2}}$$

The equation for *physiologic dead space* was given earlier.

Blood Gases and pH

O_2 dissolved in blood:

$$C_{O_2} = Sol \cdot P_{O_2}$$

where Sol is $0.003 \; ml \cdot dl^{-1} \cdot mm \; Hg^{-1}$.
  Henderson-Hasselbalch equation:

$$pH = pK_A + \log\frac{[HCO_3^-]}{[CO_2]}$$

The pK_A for this system is normally 6.1. If HCO_3^- and CO_2 concentrations are in millimoles per liter, CO_2 can be replaced by P_{CO_2} (mm Hg) $\times 0.030$.

Mechanics of Breathing

Compliance $= \Delta V / \Delta P$
  Specific compliance $= \Delta V / (\Delta P \cdot V)$
  Laplace equation for the pressure caused by the surface tension of a sphere:

$$P = \frac{2T}{r}$$

where r is the radius. Note that for a soap bubble, $P = 4T/r$ because there are two surfaces.

Poiseuille's law for laminar flow:

$$\dot{V} = \frac{P\pi r^4}{8nl}$$

where n is the coefficient of viscosity* and P is the pressure difference across the length l.
  Reynolds number:

$$Re = \frac{2rvd}{n}$$

where v is average linear velocity of the gas, d is its density, and n its viscosity.
  Pressure drop for laminar flow is $P \propto \dot{V}$, but pressure drop for turbulent flow is $P \propto \dot{V}^2$ (approximately).
  Airway resistance:

$$\frac{P_{alv} - P_{mouth}}{\dot{V}}$$

where P_{alv} and P_{mouth} refer to alveolar and mouth pressures, respectively.

Normal Values

Reference Values for Lung Function Tests

Normal values depend on age, sex, height, weight, and ethnic origin. This is a complex subject, and for a detailed discussion the reader is referred to Cotes JE. Lung function. 5th ed. Oxford: Blackwell, 1993;445–513. Reference values for some commonly used tests are shown in **TABLE A–1**. There is evidence that people are becoming healthier and that lung function is improving.

---

* This is a corruption of the Greek letter η for those of us who have little Latin and less Greek.

TABLE A–1.
Example of Reference Values for Some Commonly Used Pulmonary Function Tests in White Nonsmoking Adults in the United States

	Men	Women
TLC (l)	7.95 St + 0.003 A - 7.33 (0.79)	5.90 St - 4.54 (0.54)
FVC (l)	7.74 St - 0.021 A - 7.75 (0.51)	4.14 St - 0.023 A - 2.20 (0.44)
RV (l)	2.16 St + 0.021 A - 2.84 (0.37)	1.97 St + 0.020 A - 2.42 (0.38)
FRC (l)	4.72 St + 0.009 A - 5.29 (0.72)	3.60 St + 0.003 A - 3.18 (0.52)
RV/TLC (%)	0.309 A + 14.1 (4.38)	0.416 A + 14.35 (5.46)
FEV_1 (l)	5.66 St - 0.023 A - 4.91 (0.41)	2.68 St - 0.025 A - 0.38 (0.33)
FEV_1/FVC (%)	110.2 - 13.1 St - 0.15 A (5.58)	124.4 - 21.4 St - 0.15 A (6.75)
$FEF_{25-75\%}$ ($l \cdot s^{-1}$)	5.79 St - 0.036 A - 4.52 (1.08)	3.00 St - 0.031 A - 0.41 (0.85)
$MEF_{50\% \; FVC}$ ($l \cdot s^{-1}$)	6.84 St - 0.037 A - 5.54 (1.29)	3.21 St - 0.024 A - 0.44 (0.98)
$MEF_{25\% \; FVC}$ ($l \cdot s^{-1}$)	3.10 St - 0.023 A - 2.48 (0.69)	1.74 St - 0.025 A - 0.18 (0.66)
D_L ($ml \cdot min^{-1} \cdot mm \; Hg^{-1}$)	16.4 St - 0.229 A + 12.9 (4.84)	16.0 St - 0.111 A + 2.24 (3.95)
D_L/V_A	10.09 - 2.24 St - 0.031 A (0.73)	8.33 - 1.81 St - 0.016 A (0.80)

St is stature (height) (m). A is age (years). Standard deviation is in parentheses.
From Cotes JE. *Lung Function*. 5th ed. Oxford: Blackwell, 1993.

Further Reading

References for Individual Chapters

This list includes some recent reviews, classic papers, and books.

Chapter 1

Murray JF. *The Normal Lung*. 2nd ed. Philadelphia: WB Saunders, 1986.

Roughton FJW. Transport of oxygen and carbon dioxide. In: Fenn WO, Rahn H, eds. *Handbook of Physiology*, Section 3: *The Respiratory System*. Washington, DC: American Physiological Society, 1964;1:767–826.

Weibel ER. *Morphometry of the Human Lung*. New York: Academic Press, 1963.

Weibel ER. *The Pathway for Oxygen*. Cambridge: Harvard University Press, 1984.

Chapter 2

Davenport HW. *The ABC of Acid Base Chemistry*. 6th ed. Chicago: University of Chicago Press, 1974.

Hornbein TF, ed. *Regulation of Breathing*. New York: Dekker, 1981.

Rahn H, Fenn WO. *A Graphical Analysis of the Respiratory Gas Exchange. The O_2-CO_2 Diagram*. Washington, DC: American Physiological Society, 1955.

Chapter 3

Pride NB, Permutt S, Riley RL, Bromberger-Barnea B. Determinants of maximum expiratory flow from the lungs. *J Appl Physiol* 1967;23:646–662.

Rahn H, Otis AB, Chadwick LE, Fenn WO. The pressure-volume diagram of the thorax and lung. *Am J Physiol* 1946;146:161–178.

West JB. *Ventilation/Blood Flow and Gas Exchange*. 5th ed. Oxford: Blackwell, 1990.

Chapter 4

Hlastala MP. Ventilation. In: Crystal RG, West JB, Barnes PJ, Weibel ER, eds. *The Lung: Scientific Foundations*. 2nd ed. New York: Raven Press, 1997;2:1609–1614.

Paiva M. Uneven ventilation. In: Crystal RG, West JB, Barnes PJ, Weibel ER, eds. *The Lung: Scientific Foundations*. 2nd ed. New York: Raven Press, 1997;1:1403–1413.

Pedley TJ, Schroter RC, Sudlow MF. Gas flow and mixing in airways. In: West JB, ed. *Bioengineering Aspects of the Lung*. New York: Dekker, 1977:163–265.

Chapter 5

Forster RE. Diffusion of gases across the alveolar membrane. In: Farhi L, Tenney SM, eds. *Handbook of Physiology*, Section 3: *The Respiratory System*. Bethesda, MD: American Physiological Society, 1987;4:71–88.

Hoppin FG, Hildebrandt J. Mechanical properties of the lung. In: West JB, ed. *Bioengineering Aspects of the Lung*. New York: Dekker, 1977:83–162.

Scheid P, Piiper J. Diffusion. In: Crystal RG, West JB, Barnes PJ, Weibel ER, eds. *The Lung: Scientific Foundations*. 2nd ed. New York: Raven Press, 1997;2:1681–1691.

Chapter 6

Fung YC, Sobin SS. Theory of sheet flow in lung alveoli. *J Appl Physiol* 1969;26:472–488.

Glazier JB, Hughes JMB, Maloney JE, West JB. Measurements of capillary dimensions and blood volume in rapidly frozen lungs. *J Appl Physiol* 1969;26:65–76.

Permutt S, Riley RL. Hemodynamics of collapsible vessels with tone: the vascular waterfall. *J Appl Physiol* 1963;18:924–932.

Said SI. *The Pulmonary Circulation and Acute Lung Injury*. Mount Kisco, NY: Futura, 1991.

Silverman ES, Gerritsen ME, Collins T. Metabolic functions of the pulmonary endothelium. In: Crystal RG, West JB, Barnes PJ, Weibel ER, eds. *The Lung: Scientific Foundations*. 2nd ed. New York: Raven Press, 1997;1:629–651.

Chapter 7

Staub NC. The pathophysiology of pulmonary edema. *Hum Pathol* 1970;1:419–432.

Taylor AE, Khimenko PL, Moore TM, Adkins WK. Fluid balance. In: Crystal RG, West JB, Barnes PJ, Weibel ER, eds. *The Lung: Scientific Foundations.* 2nd ed. New York: Raven Press, 1997;2:1549–1566.

Chapter 8

Gonda I. Particle deposition in the human respiratory tract. In: Crystal RG, West JB, Barnes PJ, Weibel ER, eds. *The Lung: Scientific Foundations.* 2nd ed. New York: Raven Press, 1997;2:2289–2294.

Heppleston AG, Leopold JG. Chronic pulmonary emphysema: anatomy and pathogenesis. *Am J Med* 1961;31:279–291.

Ulmer WT, Reichel G. Functional impairment in coal worker's pneumoconiosis. *Ann NY Acad Sci* 1972; 200:405–412.

Chapter 9

Bone RC, George RB, Hudson LD. *Acute Respiratory Failure.* New York: Churchill Livingstone, 1987.

Canonico AE, Brigham KL. Biology of acute injury. In: Crystal RG, West JB, Barnes PJ, Weibel ER, eds. *The Lung: Scientific Foundations.* 2nd ed. New York: Raven Press, 1997;2:2475–2498.

General Reference Texts

Physiology

The sections on physiology in this book are based on my book, *Respiratory Physiology—The Essentials.* 6th ed. Baltimore: Lippincott Williams & Wilkins, 2000. More details on some of the topics can be found in that book.

For an exhaustive treatment of most aspects of respiratory physiology, see the five volumes of Fishman AP, ed. *Handbook of Physiology*, Section 3: *The Respiratory System.* Bethesda, MD: American Physiological Society, 1986.

Another useful source for detailed physiology is Crystal RG, West JB, Barnes PJ, Weibel ER, eds. *The Lung: Scientific Foundations.* 2nd ed. New York: Raven Press, 1997.

Pathophysiology

The sections on pathophysiology are based on my book, *Pulmonary Pathophysiology—The Essentials.* 5th ed. Baltimore: Lippincott Williams & Wilkins, 1998. That book has more information on some of the topics covered here.

Reference texts for additional material include (1) Crystal RG, West JB, Barnes PJ, Weibel ER, eds. *The Lung: Scientific Foundations.* 2nd ed. New York: Raven Press, 1997, and (2) Murray JF, Nadel JA, Mason RB, Boushey HA, eds. *Textbook of Respiratory Medicine.* 3rd ed. Philadelphia: WB Saunders, 2000.

Clinical Medicine

Good reference textbooks include (1) Murray JF, Nadel JA, Mason RB, Boushey HA, eds. *Textbook of Respiratory Medicine.* 3rd ed. Philadelphia: WB Saunders, 2000, and (2) standard textbooks of medicine such as Fauci AS, et al., eds. *Harrison's Principles of Internal Medicine.* 14th ed. New York: McGraw-Hill, 1998, and Bennett JC, Plum F, eds. *Cecil Textbook of Medicine.* 20th ed. Philadelphia: WB Saunders, 1996.

Anatomy

There are good chapters on morphology in Crystal RG, West JB, Barnes PJ, Weibel ER, eds. *The Lung: Scientific Foundations.* 2nd ed. New York: Raven Press, 1997. Excellent drawings of anatomy can be found in Netter FP. *Ciba Collection of Medical Illustrations.* West Caldwell, NJ: Ciba Pharmaceutical Products, 1993.

Pathology

Appropriate chapters of Crystal RG, West JB, Barnes PJ, Weibel ER, eds. *The Lung: Scientific Foundations.* 2nd ed. New York: Raven Press, 1997. Another good standard textbook of pathology is Cotran RS, Kumar V, Collins T. *Robbins Pathologic Basis of Disease.* 6th ed. Philadelphia: WB Saunders, 1999.

Appendix C

Answers to Questions

Chapter 1

1. C
2. E
3. D
4. B
5. C
6. C
7. D
8. E

Chapter 2

1. B
2. B
3. E
4. E
5. D
6. C
7. E
8. D
9. A
10. C
11. E
12. C

Chapter 3

1. B
2. D
3. D
4. C
5. D
6. A
7. D
8. E
9. E
10. E

Chapter 4

1. E
2. E
3. D
4. D
5. D
6. B
7. E
8. C

Chapter 5

1. D
2. B
3. D
4. A
5. D
6. B
7. E
8. A

Chapter 6

1. B
2. C
3. A
4. E
5. B
6. E
7. C
8. B
9. E
10. C
11. A
12. E
13. D

Chapter 7

1. B
2. B
3. A
4. B
5. D
6. E
7. E
8. A

Chapter 8

1. D
2. C
3. E
4. D
5. E
6. D
7. E
8. B
9. E

Chapter 9

1. B
2. C
3. E
4. B
5. B
6. D
7. E
8. D
9. C

Figure and Table Credits

Figure 1–5. Modified from Weibel ER: *The Pathway for Oxygen.* Cambridge: Harvard University Press, 1984, p 275.

Figure 1–6. Modified from West JB: *Ventilation/Blood Flow and Gas Exchange,* ed 5. Oxford: Blackwell, 1990, p 3.

Figure 1–7. Modified from Weibel ER: Morphological basis of alveolar-capillary gas exchange. *Physiol Rev* 53:419–495, 1973.

Figure 1–11. Reproduced with permission from Maloney JE, Castle BL: Pressure-diameter relations of capillaries and small blood vessels in frog lung. *Respir Physiol* 7:150–162, 1969.

Figure 1–12. Reproduced with permission from Glazier JB, Hughes JM, Maloney JE, West JB: Measurements of capillary dimensions and blood volume in rapidly frozen lungs. *J Appl Physiol* 26:65–76, 1969.

Figure 2–8. Reproduced with permission from Nielsen M, Smith H: *Acta Physiol Scand* 24:293–313, 1951.

Figure 2–10. Modified from Hurtado A: In Dill DB: *Handbook of Physiology, Adaptation to the Environment.* Washington, DC: American Physiological Society, 1964.

Figure 3–4. Modified from Thurlbeck WM: *Chronic Airflow Obstruction in Lung Disease.* Philadelphia: Saunders, 1976.

Figure 3–5. Reproduced with permission from Thurlbeck WM: *Chronic Airflow Obstruction in Lung Disease.* Philadelphia: Saunders, 1976.

Figure 3–11. Reproduced with permission from West JB: *Ventilation/Blood Flow and Gas Exchange,* ed 5. Oxford: Blackwell, 1990.

Figure 3–12. Reproduced with permission from West JB: *Ventilation/Blood Flow and Gas Exchange,* ed 5. Oxford: Blackwell, 1990.

Figure 3–15. Redrawn from Fry DL, Hyatt RE: *Am J Med* 29:672–679, 1960.

Figure 3–17. Reproduced with permission from West JB: *Ventilation/Blood Flow and Gas Exchange,* ed 5. Oxford: Blackwell, 1990.

Figure 3–18. Reproduced with permission from West JB: *Ventilation/Blood Flow and Gas Exchange,* ed 5. Oxford: Blackwell, 1990.

Figure 3–20. Reproduced with permission from West JB: *Lancet* 2:1055–1058, 1963.

Figure 3–21. Modified from West JB: *Ventilation/Blood Flow and Gas Exchange,* ed 5. Oxford: Blackwell, 1990.

Figure 3–22. Redrawn from Wagner PD, Laravuso RB, Uhl RR, West JB: Continuous distributions of ventilation-perfusion ratios in normal subjects breathing air and 100 per cent O_2. *J Clin Invest* 54:54–68, 1974.

Figure 3–23. Reproduced with permission from Wagner PD, Dantzker DR, Dueck R, *et al*: Ventilation-perfusion inequality in chronic obstructive pulmonary disease. *J Clin Invest* 59:203–216, 1977.

Figure 4–2. Modified from Bates DV, *et al*: *Respiratory Function in Disease,* ed 2. Philadelphia: Saunders, 1971.

Figure 4–4. Modified from Bates DV, *et al*: *Respiratory Function in Disease,* ed 2. Philadelphia: Saunders, 1971.

Figure 4–10. Redrawn from Pedley TJ, Schroter RC, Sudlow MF: The prediction of pressure drop and variation of resistance within the human bronchial airways. *Respir Physiol* 9:387–405, 1970.

Figure 5–2. Reproduced with permission from Hinson KFW: Diffuse pulmonary fibrosis. *Hum Pathol* 1:275–288, 1970.

Figure 5–3. Reproduced with permission from Weibel ER, Gil J: In West JB (ed): *Bioengineering Aspects of the Lung.* New York: Marcel Dekker, 1977.

Figure 5–4. Modified from Gracey DR, Divertie MB, Brown AL Jr: Alveolar-capillary membrane in idiopathic interstitial pulmonary fibrosis. Electron microscopic study of 14 cases. *Am Rev Respir Dis* 98:16–21, 1968.

Figure 6–6. Redrawn from Hughes JM, Glazier JB, Maloney JE, West JB: Effect of lung volume on the distribution of pulmonary blood flow in man. *Respir Physiol* 4:58–72, 1968.

Figure 6–7. Reproduced with permission from West JB, *et al*: *J Appl Physiol* 19:713–724, 1964.

Figure 6–12. Reproduced with permission from Radford EP: In Remington JW (ed): *Tissue Elasticity.* Washington, DC: American Physiological Society, 1957.

Figure 7–4. Reproduced with permission from Staub NC: The pathophysiology of pulmonary edema. *Hum Pathol* 1:419–432, 1970.

Figure 8–5. Reproduced with permission from Heppleston AG, Leopold JG: *Am J Med* 31:279–291, 1961.

Figure 8–8. Reproduced with permission from Ulmer WT, Reichel G: Functional impairment in coal workers' pneumoconiosis. *Ann N Y Acad Sci* 200:405–412, 1972.

Figure 9–2. Reproduced with permission from Lamy M, Fallat RJ, Koeniger E, *et al*: Pathologic features and mechanisms of hypoxemia in adult respiratory distress syndrome. *Am Rev Respir Dis* 114:267–284, 1976.

Figure 9–6. Modified from Kapanci Y, Weibel ER, Kaplan HP, Robinson FR: Pathogenesis and reversibility of the pulmonary lesions of oxygen toxicity in monkeys. II. Ultrastructural and morphometric studies. *Lab Invest* 20:101–118, 1969.

Figure 9–12. Modified from Dantzker DR, Brook CJ, Dehart P, *et al*: Ventilation-perfusion distributions in the adult respiratory distress syndrome. *Am Rev Respir Dis* 120:1039–1052, 1979.

Figure 9–13. Reproduced with permission from Glazier JB, Hughes JM, Maloney JE, West JB: Measurements of capillary dimensions and blood volume in rapidly frozen lungs. *J Appl Physiol* 26:65–76, 1969.

Table A–1. Reproduced with permission from Cotes JE. *Lung Function*, ed 5. Oxford: Blackwell, 1993.

Index

Page numbers in *italics* denote figures; those followed by a "t" denote tables